RESTORE YOUR LOST VISION NOW

RESTORE YOUR LOST VISION NOW

THE THREE-STEP PROGRAM TO *REGAIN* YOUR SIGHT

DENNIS J. COURTNEY, MD

Advantage

Copyright © 2016 by Dennis J. Courtney, MD.

All rights reserved. No part of this book may be used or reproduced in any manner whatsoever without prior written consent of the author, except as provided by the United States of America copyright law.

Published by Advantage, Charleston, South Carolina.
Member of Advantage Media Group.

ADVANTAGE is a registered trademark and the Advantage colophon is a trademark of Advantage Media Group, Inc.

Printed in the United States of America.

ISBN: 978-1-59932-772-3
LCCN: 2016953992

Cover design by Katie Biondo.

This publication is designed to provide accurate and authoritative information in regard to the subject matter covered. It is sold with the understanding that the publisher is not engaged in rendering legal, accounting, or other professional services. If legal advice or other expert assistance is required, the services of a competent professional person should be sought.

Advantage Media Group is proud to be a part of the Tree Neutral® program. Tree Neutral offsets the number of trees consumed in the production and printing of this book by taking proactive steps such as planting trees in direct proportion to the number of trees used to print books. To learn more about Tree Neutral, please visit **www.treeneutral.com**.

Advantage Media Group is a publisher of business, self-improvement, and professional development books. We help entrepreneurs, business leaders, and professionals share their Stories, Passion, and Knowledge to help others Learn & Grow. Do you have a manuscript or book idea that you would like us to consider for publishing? Please visit **advantagefamily.com** or call 1.866.775.1696.

This book is dedicated to my beloved wife and to our four sons Joseph, Vincent, Jack, and Dennis Jr. Her early departure from this earth, although lamented, does not prevent our family from the daily celebration of her vibrant contributions to all of us. She remains constantly in our thoughts, as well as a guiding force with each passing day and forever.

TABLE OF CONTENTS

1 | **CHAPTER 1**: *Where We Are*

19 | **CHAPTER 2**: *Can This Program Work for Me?*

25 | **CHAPTER 3**: *The Retinal Diseases*

43 | **CHAPTER 4**: *Let's Take a Step Backward for a Moment*

67 | **CHAPTER 5**: *The Pledge and the Plan*

85 | **CHAPTER 6**: *The Three-Step Program to Regain Your Sight*

119 | **CHAPTER 7**: *Removing Your Toxicities*

139 | **CHAPTER 8**: *Optimize Perfusion*

165 | **CHAPTER 9**: *Getting Back to Keeping It Simple*

177 | **CHAPTER 10**: *Where Do We Go from Here?*

191 | **RESOURCES**

CHAPTER 1

WHERE WE ARE

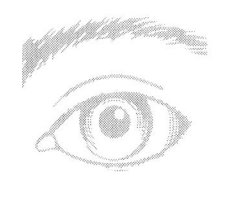

You are about to begin a journey that, unfortunately, you are not properly prepared for. You are not prepared because you have continually been told that nothing can be done to restore whatever vision you may have lost already. It is actually worse than that. You have also been told that nothing can be done to alter the further progression of the disease that is responsible for your vision loss.

Your very nice eye doctor, who is well trained in all matters concerning the eyes and the expert that you have entrusted to advise you about your vision, is quite resolute. He is concerned about you and your vision. If there were something he could do, he would do it. Yet there is no information he is prepared to discuss that even remotely suggests you will emerge with your sight intact ever again.

At this point, I want to be sure to elaborate a statement I will be repeating frequently. My intention is to provide you with the hopes and aspirations concerning your eye disease that your eye doctor has never been able to discuss with you, so here goes.

"Eighty-five to ninety percent of all patients who complete the Three-Step Program to regain their sight will have a substantial improvement in their vision in three days."

This statement accurately represents the results that have been experienced over the last ten years of offering the program throughout the United States by its originator, Dr. Edward Kondrot.

Dr. Kondrot is a board certified ophthalmologist who had a thriving practice in conventional ophthalmology with a full complement of all the surgical procedures that are expected to be performed by all eye doctors. He clearly enjoyed the years that were spent helping patients optimize their vision with the surgical skill he had developed.

He also vividly recalls having to consult with patients he could not help. All too often, he was the individual who had to tell his patients that their particular eye disorder was unable to be arrested and that the vision that was lost would not be returning. In fact, it more than likely would become worse. He became, all too frequently, the professional who had to tell the patient that "nothing can be done."

This bitter pill was an extremely difficult one to swallow, so instead he decided to develop a nonconventional program that was able to allow patients to restore their lost vision. He was only able to accomplish this by completely abandoning his ophthalmological training in how to approach these patients to restore vision that had been lost.

It should be reemphasized that for such a program to be successful, he would have to ignore everything he was taught to use from his previous medical training as an ophthalmologist if he was going to be able to revive nonfunctioning eye tissue back to functioning tissue once again.

An additional point of emphasis will also need to be that you abandon what you have learned are the limitations of medical care. You too will be required to appreciate what is possible to optimize your health.

There is a way to recapture the ability of the tissues of the human body to return to a level of functioning of an earlier period of your life. You can become vibrant and have an enthusiasm for life once again. Your unsteady gait can be supplanted by a youthful step and stride. Your weakened and aging heart and blood vessels can return to provide a healthy blood flow to all regions of the body that have slowly eroded but can function optimally once again.

Yes, if your vision has deteriorated to the point that you can no longer drive a motor vehicle or just appreciate the smiling faces of your grandchildren, your vision can be restored. That restoration can occur now.

GETTING A FRESH START

I intend to describe the abysmal and embarrassing medical model that guides your current treatment by your eye doctor. I will do so to allow you to appreciate why your doctor cannot be expected to do anything but fail in treating all chronic diseases and the diseases that are associated with advancing age.

To be able to appreciate "how you can restore your lost vision—now," it will be helpful if you can begin to appreciate the common fallacy that provides the underpinning for the recipe for failure. That fallacy is embodied by the trite and damning phrase that I feel has been used all too often: **"Nothing can be done."**

This is the phrase that signals that the ball game is over and never to be resumed again. It packs the wallop of a full blow to the gut. It is almost impossible from which to recuperate. After all, we are talking about your health, hearing, or vision.

That decree is coming from an individual to whom you have given a great degree of trust and reliance. You figure if it is coming from your doctor who knows you so well, it has to be true because he would never say such a thing if it were not the case. From that point forward, you are beaten. You are mortally wounded. You will remain devastated for as long as that phrase remains operational.

If we are to be successful in restoring your vision, the use of this phrase can no longer be tolerated and must be rejected. You can and should reject it because it is, first and foremost, not true. It, in fact, is absolutely and blatantly false.

To assist you in this rejection, allow me to qualify what your current eye doctor really means to say. Please allow me some literary latitude, and I believe the error that your doctor has committed will readily become clear.

This is what your doctor really should have said, and if he would have said it in this way, it would be 100 percent accurate.

> *Dear Mr. ____, your eye disease is one of the most common causes of vision loss, especially in the population of those patients with advancing age. Now, the disease may be common, but the ability to successfully treat it at this time is not possible. With all my training and experience and all the treatment options I have at my disposal, "nothing can be done" to correct your vision loss and/or alter the further progression of your disease.*

The accuracy of this hypothetical conversation between a doctor and his patient lies in the use of the words "and all the treatment options that I have at my disposal." This qualifying explanation illuminates why a conventionally trained ophthalmologist is destined to fail in the treatment of certain eye diseases because all his training has been centered on his treatment arsenal of surgery, procedures, and drugs.

The skills of a surgeon, the performance of procedures, and the use of certain pharmaceutical agents can be quite helpful in certain medical conditions and eye disorders. It must be said, however, that as long as the tools used by the eye doctor remain one of or multiple combinations of the prior three treatment options, the correction of serious eye diseases that can lead to blindness cannot possibly ever be conquered.

The problem does not lie within the intention and intelligence of the brilliant members of the medical profession. The problem lies within the tools available to these professionals, which are woefully inadequate to revive diseased eye tissue and allow it to function once again.

The point I believe I should make here is that in the Three-Step Program to restore your vision, there is no surgery. There are no procedures. There are no drugs to be used. Instead, as you will see, there are modalities and nondrug therapies that will revive dysfunctional eye tissue back to function once again.

Legitimate questions can be raised for how it can be that the medical profession in general and the specialty of ophthalmology in particular do not have the proper tools to reverse eye diseases. What is even more pathetic is that the conventional medical community is devoid and absent of any knowledge of the therapies that have demonstrated the ability to reverse the eye disease process and return function to dysfunctional eye tissue.

You can restore your lost vision—now. You can begin that process by immediately putting in play the therapies and modalities we will present here.

I emphasize, however, if there is one thing you can do to initiate this return of function, it is to dismiss as false the notion that "nothing can be done," no matter who the individual was that proposed the idea to begin with. I mention again that "85 to 90 percent of all patients who complete this Three-Step Program to return their sight will have a substantial improvement in their vision in three days."

INTEGRATIVE MEDICINE–IT IS JUST DIFFERENT

I have had the opportunity to consult with thousands of patients over the many years I have been in the practice of integrative medicine. On our first meeting, it becomes obvious to those individuals who consult with me that my approach to their medical issues is in stark contrast to those they have become accustomed to with their conventional medical doctors.

For starters, my first consult with a patient is at least an hour and a half. The vast majority of those are actually extended to two hours and sometimes even longer. It is not uncommon for a patient to comment that he or she has never had an opportunity to spend that amount of time with the doctor over the course of their entire relationship.

The truth of the matter is that your current doctor is not in control of how he can spend his time. Insurance companies and office management decide that for him and schedule him accordingly.

The standard allotment on average, per patient, is about ten minutes and no longer. To orchestrate the flow of patients in such a way that a patient will not throw a wrench into this assembly line, a large staff of nurses, technicians, and nurse practitioners are layered into your office visit to divert the expenditure of energy from the doctor and onto that ancillary staff.

If you see the doctor at all, it will be to briefly allow you to comment on what your chief complaint is at that visit and to receive a prescription given to you by his nurse to alleviate your symptoms of that day as you are escorted out the door within the time that has been predetermined.

Rest assured that if some unanticipated event should alter the flow of patient traffic, there will be a staff meeting to expose the weak link in the system, which usually signals the need to dismiss the employee who cannot keep up the pace. In this system, you cannot ever be rewarded for going above and beyond the call of duty for the benefit of patient care because that additional care takes time, and time is what dictates the success or failure of the system.

In my experience, I have observed that there are essentially three categories of patients that I have the opportunity to manage as a doctor.

Category 1: those patients who elect to pursue alternative medicine by first intention

This group of patients has chosen a course of alternative treatment as their first choice and avoids conventional medical management.

Allow me to share a story I contend is occurring with increasing regularity that will help describe a group of patients that is growing in number every year.

The patient is a fifty-five-year-old male who comes to my office and, after pleasantries are exchanged, begins to talk about his particular medical situation. In a resolute voice, he starts his summary by indicating he had been diagnosed with pancreatic cancer. He goes on to say that his preliminary diagnosis was based on a CT scan as well as a PET scan, and tissue will have to be obtained through biopsy in order to confirm that diagnosis.

At that point, he becomes quite definitive on what his course of action is going to be from this point forward. He announces that there will be no biopsy he will consent to. He also says he will not submit to any surgical intervention on his behalf. He says that chemotherapy may be indicated both before and after surgery, which he absolutely refuses. Finally, he states that he will not consent to any radiation therapy being performed upon him prior to or after a surgery would be completed.

As should be obvious the patient does not want to have anything to do with the conventional medical treatment of pancreatic cancer. He claims that he is there that day to discuss with me what alternative and integrative program may be proposed that he can pursue in order to assist in the eradication of the cancer.

It is apparent to me that he fully understands the ramifications of his decision to the extent that, in his opinion and by his choice, he is not interested in conventional therapy of any kind as one of his treatment options. He instead wishes to discuss the treatment options available to him from the alternative-medical realm, which he feels hold the best opportunity for him to have any impact on his pancreatic disease. He is attentively awaiting a description by me as to how pancreatic cancer may be treated through the integrative process.

This gentleman's situation is obviously a serious one. It does point out, however, that even in a situation where there are known therapies to pursue, there are many individuals who intuitively understand the shortcomings of conventional medicine and will not allow those shortcomings to dictate their medical course of action and medical therapies that they wish to pursue.

Numerous patients of mine come to me with other medical ailments with a far lesser degree of gravity associated with them, but the story remains the same. They select to pursue integrative and alternative approaches to their medical problems and avoid conventional therapy essentially, in their opinion, at all costs.

Each of these patients has a primary-care physician. The patients have insurance coverage that will allow them to be seen by their physicians and have their insurance reimburse that encounter. These patients, however, understand the limitations of the conventional medical model. They also understand that the use of pharmaceutical agents within that model does nothing to correct the problem for which they have sought the medical attention but instead only suppresses the symptoms that are provoked by those disorders.

Category 2: those patients who pursue alternative and integrative medicine as a last resort

This group of patients has serious medical issues for which they have consulted with a multitude of medical doctors over an extended period of time. They continue their search in the hope that the next doctor will have the key to unlock the answers that have eluded all the health practitioners they have consulted with to date.

As far as conventional doctors are concerned, they were the first arena of pursuit of these individuals. After extensive evaluations by multiple practitioners as well as multiple medical disciplines, no diagnosis that had been operational ever has solved their medical dilemma.

This group of patients, however, has not given up the hope and possibility of regaining their health again. Instead, they begin to pursue the alternative arena in the hopes that this group of professionals may find the answer to their particular medical problems.

I find these patients to be extremely knowledgeable in medical matters. They have an appreciation for multiple medical modalities that they think may be used on their behalf. They have already bought into the fact that their unhealthy tissue can be revived and restored to full function once again if only they can be guided by a medical professional to allow that to become their new reality.

They have learned on their own that even when the conventional medical community has diagnosed their problem, the treatments used in the conventional arena have not been able, nor does it appear that they ever will be able, to restore them to fully functional once again. They have therefore learned on their own that for them to function well, their tissues must be restored to normal function and that with the tools found within the conventional medical community, this will not be possible in their case.

Category 3: patients who have no options for further treatment

In this group of patients, after all conventional treatment measures have failed, the patient is then informed that no further treatment is available, in a sense providing no way to regain health and vitality ever again.

It is in this category that I find the majority of the patients who participate in our eye-treatment programs. These are the patients of the true "nothing can be done" individuals who suffer from incurable diseases that the medical profession itself has given up on.

I have consulted with many who have found themselves in such an unfortunate category of disease. It could be a cancer patient who has completed a surgery and undergone multiple rounds of chemotherapy and an equal number of radiation sessions. At some point, it is standard operating procedure to advise the patient that no further treatment is available and that he should "get his affairs in order" and await the inevitable.

A patient who comes to my care with that history does not and should not hear from me that "nothing can be done." The fact of the matter is that there is always something that can be done, and those efforts can be and are worthwhile to, at a minimum, improve their current situation and quality of life.

There is something that can be said about the members of this group of patients that actually puts them in an easier decision-making situation than is found in any of the other groups. That happens to be the undeniable situation that they really do not have any other competing therapy to even consider. If they do not choose the treatment program I offer to them, it is not as though they have any other therapy, program, or treatment option to put in its place. The true fact of the matter is there is no other therapy. There is no other treatment program. There just is not any other viable alternative except for one, which is to do nothing at all and accept the inevitable consequences of that decision.

Many patients become resigned to the fact that their disease and health are just going to continue to deteriorate. They have already had this notion confirmed by their own doctor, a person in whom they have established a great degree of trust and, for that reason, would never say "nothing more can be done" if it were not so.

Let's be clear. No doctor should ever extinguish the hopes and aspirations of getting well for any reason whatsoever. There is always something that can be done. Just because all conventional medical treatment has failed does not mean some other clinician does not have a plan to succeed where others have failed.

In reality, there is no difference between the cancer patient who is told that all treatment is suspended and that he should go home to "get his affairs in order" and the eye patient who is told by his doctor that "nothing can be done," and vision loss will continue to deteriorate. In both cases, the hope of getting better is extinguished. In a cancer patient, a life will come to an end as the ultimate consequence of the decision not to treat. The eye patient does not die due to the lack of a viable treatment option, but I will share with you that in many cases, patients have confided in me to reveal that they wish they would.

IT DOES NOT MATTER HOW YOU GET THERE

There are some patients who have greatly impressed me with their medical acumen of these complex eye disorders. They have made their eye disease their newfound life's project.

In just about all cases, these patients recalled the conversation they had with their eye doctor concerning their own treatment program and how they felt when they were told "nothing can be done." The initial impact of that encounter was not necessarily painful in a physical way but was psychologically lethal beyond description. The recovery time from that event varies.

One thing tends to be a common link among them all: from that point forward, they will find a solution to their eye dilemma. They will never forget that meeting with their eye doctor, and they view finding the solution as a very personal mission. In pursuit of that mission, failure is not an option.

There are other patients who just happen to stumble across our eye programs. A relative or friend tells them to check out our practice. They just happen to come across information about our practice. Someone just hands them some of our literature or our advertisement.

With minimal effort, we have a chance to meet and describe the eye-treatment program in great depth. After the explanation is concluded, it is then that many of the questions emerge that provide the clues that suggest the patient really has a difficult time believing what I am telling them is true. It is helpful for you to hear some of those commonly asked questions that test the boundaries of incredulity and the simple responses that follow.

The point I would like to make is that it does not matter how you arrive here, whether you are the informed patient on a mission to regain your sight or the patient who abruptly learns there is medical help available to regain your vision. I think you already know the consequence of a decision to do nothing at all and where that ultimately may bring you with your sight.

This book and this eye program are intended to allow you to take charge of your medical and visual future and remove the option of doing nothing at all as unacceptable.

The following chapters of this book will concentrate on a detailed explanation of how you can restore your lost vision. Only the reader will be able to determine if these answers are sufficient enough to encourage them to participate in the modalities and therapies we describe.

The best area of focus to anyone with lingering doubt is the results that have been experienced over the last ten to twelve years from those who have completed the program. Those results should be the guiding force in the determination of whether or not to participate in the Three-Step Program.

It ultimately continues to come down to one salient point, which is "85 to 90 percent of all patients who complete the Three-Step Program will have a substantial improvement in their vision."

Now we can and will discuss what is meant by the word "substantial." For now, the reader's attention should not be on how much improvement a participant can achieve but rather the unavoidable conclusion that a patient can obtain any improvement at all.

Up until now, you have been told and believed "nothing can be done" to restore your vision at all. If that truly were the case, why would it be possible to offer a treatment program at all to restore your sight? The answer will really only be how much restoration and how quickly that restoration can come, which will be the variable from one patient to another. If you ever can come to agree any level of visual function has improved, you have already made the case for the accuracy of the claim that you can restore your lost vision now.

I will be explaining how you can reverse and revive diseased eye tissue in great issues raised by patients over the course of consulting with them. I have decided that, in this case, I intend to post those questions at the beginning of the book to allow some framework to understand what those questions may be way before the answers ever become obvious to you.

It would be my fondest desire that none of these questions would even be necessary if, after having read the book, you were fully comfortable with the Three-Step Program to restore your vision. If, in fact, this book does its job in the manner I wish it to be done, that actually may happen.

The greater likelihood is there will be questions. Quite honestly, there should be questions. I am presenting a few of those right now to you to provide you with a little peek of what is coming up in the future and laying some groundwork that may actually be descriptive of your own personal eye issue and may reveal questions you would have likely asked at the conclusion of the book anyway.

Question 1: My eye doctor tells me there is no treatment for my eye disease. How can you say there is?

Answer: The three-day treatment program was developed by Dr. Edward Kondrot, a board certified ophthalmologist from Western Pennsylvania. Dr.

Kondrot was an accomplished ophthalmologist and eye surgeon who had a completely conventional practice in the treatment of all eye diseases early in his career. Dr. Kondrot was quite successful in that practice and performed all the surgeries expected of him by his patients and did so quite effectively.

A little-known fact about Dr. Kondrot is that he had a serious condition of asthma and was being consulted by medical personnel for it. He had the opportunity and ability to seek medical advice from the best lung doctors and allergy physicians in the Western Pennsylvania area. With all that medical input, Dr. Kondrot's asthma continued to worsen. Episodes of his asthmatic attacks actually increased instead of decreased.

It was at that point that Dr. Kondrot was exposed to homeopathy to determine if there could be a therapy that would be helpful for his asthma. In fact, Dr. Kondrot had his condition of asthma cured through the use of homeopathy. Because of that, he began to become attracted to the use of alternative medicine to be included in his ophthalmological practice.

This ultimately led to Dr. Kondrot managing two different practices while in Western Pennsylvania. One practice, his conventionally managed practice, was located in downtown Pittsburgh. It thrived with the conventional therapies he was trained to employ. An additional practice found in the suburban area of Pittsburgh enabled Dr. Kondrot to use alternative means to correct eye disorders, especially those that did not have a surgical correction component to them.

It was not too long before Dr. Kondrot could easily determine that the patients in his alternative eye practice were doing much better than any of his patients suffering from similar conditions found in his conventional practice.

It was at that point that Dr. Kondrot made a decision to withdraw himself from conventional ophthalmology. He moved his practice to Phoenix, Arizona, and spent a number of years developing the well-known three-day Kondrot Eye Program during that period.

Once the program was fully developed, he traveled throughout the United States offering that Three-Day Program in various cities throughout the country, enabling those afflicted with eye disorders in those regions to obtain the expertise of the three-day treatment program to restore their vision.

I mention all this information concerning Dr. Kondrot because he is the originator of it. Other ophthalmologists trained in conventional therapies have no understanding or awareness of the Kondrot Program. All the modalities used within the program are unique to alternative medicine and are never found in the conventional form of medicinal care.

Your eye doctor has told you that "nothing can be done" because, from his viewpoint and his therapies, your disease does not have a treatment that allows him to be successful in reversing it. Dr. Kondrot, through the use of the alternative approaches he incorporates within the program, actually is able to restore vision because he can revive this nonfunctioning tissue to levels of functioning eye tissue once again.

Your eye doctor is accurate. From his perspective and training, no treatment exists to restore your lost vision. It is only through the Dr. Kondrot approach using alternative measures that this becomes possible and viable with respect to your particular eye problem.

Question 2: How does the program work, and what do you do?

Answer: Day one consists of an eye examination and assessment performed by both myself as well as a professional optometrist to determine your exact eye status at the time you begin the program. Then in the ensuing three days, there is an aggressive treatment regime starting at nine o'clock in the morning and ending at four o'clock in the afternoon each day, allowing patients to receive a multitude of alternative modalities with the intention of restoring function to dysfunctional tissue.

On the third day, at the conclusion of those aggressive therapies, reassessments occur to document how much improvement patients have gained in their vision as a result of the three-day treatment program. They then return home able to perform all those modalities daily, allowing them to improve to an even greater level of functioning than they demonstrated at the time the program had been completed.

The end result of these measures is to maximize a patient's vision over that time period and restore the lost vision that had necessitated the program to begin with.

Question 3: My eye doctor has me taking medications for my eyes. What should I do about those medicines?

Answer: Dr. Kondrot and I both feel very strongly about not interfering with your relationship with your own ophthalmologist. Your eye doctor has developed a relationship with you that should be maintained, and you should continue consulting with your eye doctor when you return home. You should continue whatever medications your eye doctor has prescribed, only allowing him to decide if and when the medications may not be necessary to take anymore.

It is not uncommon for eye doctors to discover that the improvement in their patient's vision is to such an extent that the medicines previously prescribed by them are no longer necessary or, at a minimum, can be reduced substantially. It is for this reason that we do not interfere with your current medications and advise you to take them as your eye doctor has prescribed.

Question 4: My eye condition is referred to as macular degeneration and has been called a wet form of the disease. I am currently receiving injections by my

eye doctor for that condition. Can I avoid these eye injections by doing the Three-Day Program?

Answer: The form of macular degeneration that you have, which is known as wet macular degeneration, is characterized by bleeding within the retina of the eye. It is an acceptable medical procedure to require injecting these bleeding areas with a substance that will stop all hemorrhaging from occurring. If your eye doctor feels that you need to have these injections, it is his professional opinion we want you to follow, and we will rely on him to make that decision in your best medical interest.

I will say that injections need to be considered as a last resort and never a first option. Because of this, if you have been recommended to have those eye injections and you are concerned about receiving them, it is appropriate to attempt the three-day treatment program to see if the injection actually is necessary at all.

There have been many patients who have come to the eye program, with their doctors having advised them to have the injections, only to discover that the injections were not necessary by the conclusion of the Three-Day Program.

Once again, a relationship with your own eye doctor needs to be maintained and intact. We will rely completely on your eye doctor's assessment of your medical status to make that decision.

Question 5: I am interested in participating in your three-day eye program. I would like to discuss the program with my own eye doctor to find out what he thinks about it. I am scheduled to see him in a week for a regular checkup. I will make a decision concerning future participation in your program after I have spoken to him.

Answer: I certainly do not mind any dialogue you may develop concerning your eye care with your own eye doctor. I will say that it will be unfair for your eye doctor to comment about a program that he has never been exposed to or studied in his medical career.

There are a couple of points I think you should keep in mind in making a final decision. The first of these points is that the treatment approaches used during our program can present no harm to you whatsoever. They do not involve drugs, surgery, or medical procedures.

Second, to the best of my knowledge, there is no other program that has the ability to restore your lost vision. That certainly includes all the medical modalities used by your eye doctor on your behalf.

You should take your time making your ultimate decision. In my opinion, that decision should rest with you and in consulting with people who have training equal to my own, are skilled in the use of alternative therapies, and may be actually able to provide some input of value to that decision-making process.

CHAPTER 2

CAN THIS PROGRAM WORK FOR ME?

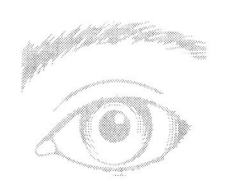

Having completed a discussion that has pledged to rescue your vision, it seems appropriate to be specific about the eye conditions that have demonstrated the greatest likelihood to achieve that success. It is for that reason that I will take the opportunity to become highly specific about the eye conditions that respond to the Three-Step Program the best.

Before turning to those specifics, some revealing generalities are in order. The first of these generalities is actually completely opposite of what you might think. In reality, there are certain eye conditions treated quite successfully by conventional approaches that result in optimizing your sight so well that it would be difficult to develop an alternative treatment program that could do better.

A good example of this group of patients would be those who suffer from diseases of the cornea. Many procedures performed with or without laser intervention have the capacity to reshape the cornea and allow the vast majority of those patients to achieve 20/20 vision without the need for glasses or contact lenses. The surgical expertise demonstrated by these eye professionals is highly commendable, and the patients who benefit from that skill are quite appreciative of their efforts.

It should be pointed out that the cornea of the eye is quite amenable to surgical intervention in which the shape of that structure can be altered to allow it to be "reshaped." With that reshaping completed, the cornea can have all its distortions corrected and, by doing so, permit flawless refraction of light to focus with precision on the retina.

To demonstrate even greater domination of this group of eye disorders by conventional means, if all else fails, ophthalmologists can elect to completely remove the cornea and replace it with a donated cadaver cornea through transplantation.

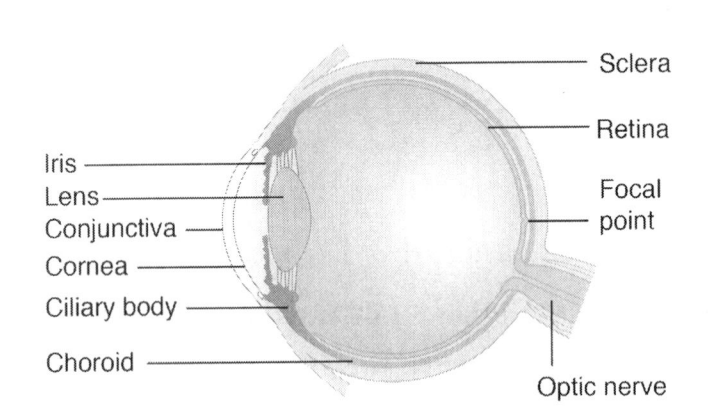

The take-home message for public consumption is as follows: most, if not all, corneal diseases can be corrected. Vision can and will be restored. How wonderful and consoling that must be for those afflicted with corneal dysfunction.

Before becoming too laudatory about how well the ophthalmology profession is able to deal with difficult visual problems, it will serve the conversation well to point out a group of eye diseases they are not able to treat well at all. In fact, it is this group of eye diseases that the Three-Step Program has been dedicated to resolve.

This group of disorders encompasses the eye diseases that affect the retina, which is the portion of the eye that captures the image sent to it from the lens.

That image is then converted into an electrical signal, which is sent to a portion of the brain where it can be interpreted.

Problems that alter the function of the cornea and lens can distort an image before it arrives at the retina. Nonetheless, that image can still be sent by the retina to the brain. Problems in the retina mean that no message will be sent at all to the brain. That ultimately leads to partial or total blindness.

It should be obvious that the retinal diseases are the most devastating of all eye disorders. The reason for this, according to conventional wisdom, is that unlike corneal and lens problems, which can be salvaged by sophisticated surgical intervention, no such surgical rescue is possible for diseases of the retina.

These retinal eye disorders as a group have the following things in common from the perspective of traditional medicine:

- There is no known treatment available to reverse retinal diseases.

- There is no way to slow the progression of retinal diseases. How quickly or slowly they progress is due to the uniqueness of the patient who suffers from it.

- Once retinal tissue is "lost," it can never be restored to function again.

Traditional medicine is convinced in these cases that "nothing can be done" and takes every opportunity to convey that message to their patients. You will come to understand it is with this group of patients that the success of the Three-Step Program will demonstrate quite the opposite viewpoint.

With that in mind, allow me to correct the three aforementioned clinical facts to reflect a more realistic assessment of the retinal diseases.

1. Retinal diseases are reversible.

2. Not only can the progression of a retinal disease be slowed down, but it also can actually be reversed.

3. Diseased retinal tissue can be revived to functional tissue once again and, in the process, restore vision that has been believed to be lost forever.

WHAT EYE DISEASES RESPOND BEST TO THE THREE-STEP PROGRAM?

The following eye diseases are representative of retinal disorders that are frequently seen as participants in our Three-Step Program. In every case, they have met the criteria created by conventional ophthalmology that continue to insist that "nothing can be done" to regain any vision that has been lost as a result of them.

As you read through the list, keep in mind that all these disorders, when properly treated, have enabled us to analyze the success we have experienced in working with these patients over a multiyear period of time. Because of that experience, the following statement can be made: "Eight-five to ninety percent of all patients who complete the three-day, three-step treatment program will have a substantial improvement in their vision."

The Retinal Diseases:

- ARMD (age-related macular degeneration)
    - wet ARMD
    - dry ARMD
- glaucoma
- diabetic retinopathy
- macular hole
- macular wrinkle

- macular pucker
- Stargardt's
- ischemic optic nerve disease
- retinitis pigmentosa
- histoplasmosis scarring
- iatrogenically induced scarring (secondary to macular degeneration injections)
- cone dystrophy

It does seem beneficial to take a moment to describe a number of these retinal diseases individually, because of some unique characteristics applicable to them. In pointing out these pertinent clinical issues, you will be better able to decide whether or not to consent to invasive procedures that could be considered as questionable at best.

This frequently happens when doctors lump them together into a large group of conditions they feel they cannot do anything about anyway. It is human nature to want to avoid excessive discussions with patients when the end result of that discussion does not change anything anyway.

When you actually can do something about these retinal diseases, that perspective is so antithetical to the traditional view that patients who suffer from these retinal diseases immediately become interested in the dialogue and, in many cases, wildly enthusiastic.

An even more important reason for discussing the retinal diseases is that, in some cases, surgical procedures will be recommended by ophthalmologists who claim that if the patient does not agree to the intervention, "They will go blind." This volatile comment seeks to provoke such fear that the net result in most cases is to acquiesce to the demands of the eye doctor even when legitimate questions can be raised.

If you are to successfully counter your doctor's insistence, you must have a logical plan to follow that can lead you to a decision based on fact and not emotion. It may be that you ultimately should consent to the intended surgery.

A good rule to follow is that any surgery or procedure should be considered only as a last resort, not the only resort. You just have to be educated in the other options at your disposal. You also must have a plan you can follow to allow you to make a decision you feel is the right decision for you.

It may turn out that the procedure actually becomes a necessary next step, but it also may confirm that you can avoid the procedure entirely because your status has improved so much that the procedure is no longer necessary.

It should be stated that it is never my intention to interfere with the relationship that exists between you and your eye doctor. He knows you and your eye condition better than any other person.

A point you must appreciate is that your doctor has never heard of the Three-Step Program. He does not know that our intention is to revive retinal tissue and restore vision. He thinks only that "nothing can be done" in your case and that his heroic measures to intervene surgically have always served him and his patients well.

Your situation is now different. You are about to begin a rejuvenation process of your retina to restore your vision. The old rules do not apply to you. In order to remain safe and avoid unnecessary intervention, reserve surgical and procedural recommendations made by your doctor as a last choice and not the first choice.

Allow a logical plan to guide you to your decision point. If the procedure becomes necessary, at least you know you have tried all preceding options. You can then have the procedure done with the confidence that it is your best option at that time.

CHAPTER 3

THE RETINAL DISEASES

MACULAR DEGENERATION

Macular degeneration is sometimes referred to as ARMD (Age-Related Macular Degeneration). The macula of the retina is the centermost portion of the retina. The aging process itself, as the name suggests, indicates a breakdown of this segment of the retina, the area that is most responsible for central vision as opposed to peripheral vision.

The breakdown of this tissue generally leads to the loss of central vision while maintaining vision peripherally. Seeing things directly in front of the patient becomes difficult, if not impossible. It is not uncommon to see a patient with macular degeneration frequently turning their head sideways where they can see clearly instead of facing forward where images are extremely difficult to process. Often, they are unable to recognize people or objects directly in front of them.

It has been estimated that by the age of seventy, one in five adults suffers from some degree of macular degeneration. It is the most common cause of blindness of all the diseases of the retina.

This disorder is a true representative of a disease associated with advancing age. The reason for this will become obvious in succeeding chapters. For now, it should be emphasized that effective measures can be taken to abate and reverse macular degeneration. Those patients afflicted with it are not irrevocably destined to lose their vision. It should be obvious, however, that the earlier those efforts are initiated, the greater the likelihood that vision will return sooner and more profoundly.

There are two types of macular degeneration. The most common form is known as dry ARMD. More than 90 percent of all cases are of this dry type. The other form of the disorder is known as wet ARMD. This disorder is characterized by the development of diseased blood vessels, which have the capacity to leak fluid or blood into the macula. In these cases, it is quite common for retinal specialists to inject directly into the diseased portion of the retina with drugs and attempt to decrease and/or arrest further bleeding.

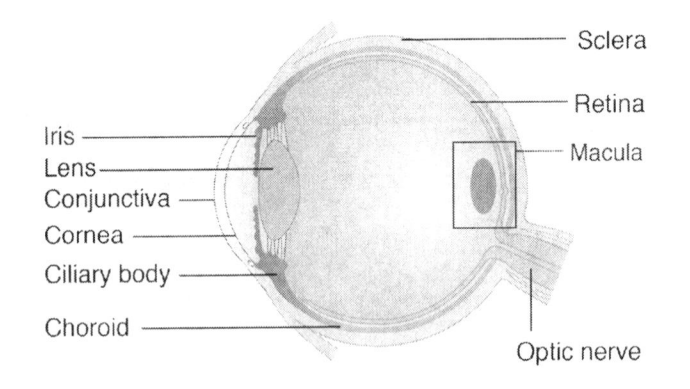

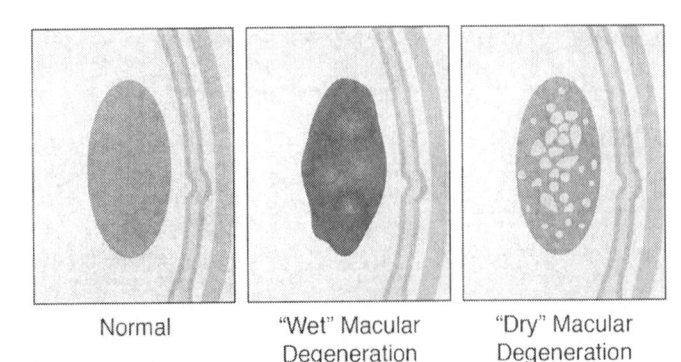

On its face value, it sounds as though it should be a good idea. The conventional literature is replete with citations that support the benefits of this type of direct intervention. If you are afflicted with wet ARMD, you must become informed about the hazards of these eye injections. There are many. In some cases, they are quite serious.

One would hope that a dutiful informed consent obtained by the doctor performing the injections would alert patients of these complications. Whether purposefully ignored or accidentally omitted, this discussion does not occur.

In the conversations I have with the majority of patients who have had the misfortune of having these anti-VEGF injections (VEGF is a hormone secreted by arteries that lead to the formation of these diseased blood vessels), they tell me they were not informed of anything detrimental that could happen as a result of receiving them. In fact, they describe what they felt their doctor essentially told them amounted to "It's either have the injection or go blind." It was expected that they would receive not just the first injection but as many in the future that the eye doctor determined to be necessary.

Very few patients with wet ARMD ever raise an objection or even hesitate to consider some other course of action. They also confide to me that they dread their next appointment with their eye doctor because of the likelihood that each visit will lead to their all-too-"automatic" next injection.

It is not my intention to interfere with the relationship between a doctor and his patient as to whether or not to pursue a treatment option proposed by him. It is apparent to me, however, that this situation is completely out of hand.

It would be a disservice not to honestly explore a logical approach as to whether or not anti-VEGF injections should be considered. This logical approach would then permit the patient to feel as though they are actually a part of their overall management, that their opinions and concerns actually will be listened to, that they actually decide what their treatment will be, that they actually have the right to refuse the injections, and, if need be, that they are justified in terminating their relationship with their current eye doctor in search for another. It also means they should consent to the injections if all other options do not produce the desired result.

The first point to be introduced is that eye patients with wet ARMD, or for that matter any retinal disease, are always placed in a defensive position. That position has only one objective: to minimize the future loss of their vision. If loss is their only motivation, they will continue to grasp at the only option presented to them by their eye doctor who is quite adamant about declaring, "You either have the injection or go blind." How can you argue or even have any discussion with your doctor after having been presented with that ultimatum?

What makes that situation even worse is that from all his training and experience, he is actually correct. He is the one working from the "nothing-can-be-done" premise I mentioned earlier. He does not know anything about a "three-day," "three-step," or for that matter a twenty-step program to turn your eye disease around and begin the process of restoring your vision.

He does not know about that possibility today, and he will not know about it tomorrow. He will not even know about it after your eye function actually returns. It makes no sense to think that your success will do anything more than confuse him. What will emerge from your education will be the formation of a strong and confident attitude concerning your health choices. Your doctors had better become ready for a new you. You are no longer fearful. You are no longer defense oriented or worried about further vision losses. You are now on offense, and you are a force to be reckoned with.

ABOUT THOSE INJECTIONS

To start your education in the right direction, there must be an honest presentation of anti-VEGF. It is only becoming apparent with more recent investigation of this procedure that serious issues have finally been correctly identified and documented by large university studies.

I want to reference a study led by Juan E. Grunwald of the University of Pennsylvania involving 1,024 patients that was known as the CATT study, (Comparison of Age-Related Macular Degeneration Treatment Trials).

All patients participating in the study were assessed prior to receiving anti-VEGF injections and, at that time, did not show any signs of a serious condition known as global atrophy (GA). Global atrophy is an area of dead and unrevivable tissue. When present, it signifies an area of the retina that does not possess any ability to function and will not ever be able to function again.

After two years of treatment, these patients were evaluated again with particular attention paid to the status of the retina where the injections were administered. Of the 1,024 patients who received anti-VEGF injections, 197 had developed global atrophy where it previously had not existed, and it was in the same area where the anti-VEGF injections had been placed.

This statistically represents 18.3 percent of the study group. This is a devastating fact that cannot be ignored in the current environment of what I observe as the flagrant use of injection therapy in wet ARMD patients.

Oddly enough, I do not see any evidence that this study and others like it have even registered a blip of concern on the radar screen of the ophthalmology profession. These professionals are doing as many injections now as they had done previously.

Global atrophy is the moribund sign that death of the retina has finally occurred. A bleeding retina is still alive, just not functioning well enough to provide a visual image. To the ophthalmologist, who does not conceive of that portion of the eye ever being able to function again, this behavior is as though retinal bleeding is a nuisance that with enough injections will just go away.

Those of us in the business of restoring function and reviving tissue vitality lament the area of global atrophy that has been provoked by the use of anti-VEGF injections. This bleeding region had the potential to function again, but as a result of the injection, which may lead to global atrophy, it never will function again.

It is an odd turn of events, which started with a doctor telling his patient, "Either have the injection or go blind." In fact, in the final analysis, approximately 20 percent of the patients who receive them actually went blind precisely because of the injection.

One additional point should be made concerning the University of Pennsylvania study. Built into the study is a blatant admission of how poorly the participants are expected to respond to the injections even when they do not experience global atrophy of the retina.

According to the criteria that was used to assess patients after the two-year study was completed, patients were allowed to demonstrate a loss in visual acuity of up to fifteen letters, which translates into three full lines of vision loss, and yet still be considered a completely successful response to the injection.

This "fudge factor" of three full lines of vision loss highlights how putrid retinal injections are and how absurd the standards for assessing them have become. These patients were already losing their vision. It appears as though the study, by design, was set up as a scenario to paint a rosy picture of acceptable vision loss when, in actuality, these results are quite candidly disastrous.

In the Three-Step Program we will be discussing, if any patient would lose as many as three letters of vision acuity, it would be considered by both the patient and me to be a failure. I can honestly say that in the time I have been offering the program, no such loss in vision has ever occurred.

The final point that needs to be made concerning the medical community's understanding of patients suffering from wet ARMD is that it is apparent to them that these patients are on a glide path to losing their sight. What remains unknown is whether the disease process progresses rapidly or slowly.

What should also be apparent is that the specialty of ophthalmology does not have any meaningful way to intervene in the process. It should be coming crystal clear that retinal injections do not change the inescapable conclusion that, at best, they do nothing and, at worst, hasten the progression of disease and accelerate the degradation process.

If that is the case, why does this professional pull out the heavyweight threat, "If you do not get these injections, you will go blind"? This is both unfair and inaccurate. It almost always leads to complete acquiescence on the part of a patient to submit to the injections to avoid the alternative predicted by the doctor.

If these injections were a solitary "one and done" situation, it may even be something to consider. What unfortunately has to be pointed out is that these patients are seen in follow-up once a month. At each succeeding doctor visit, they will more than likely receive another and yet another injection.

Finally, the vision loss will be so fulminant that the patient will be blind. It will be argued by the eye doctor that he diligently attempted to prevent it from happening, but unfortunately the disease was so progressive that even with all his best efforts to the contrary, in the end, the disease won. It will never be known for sure what brought the battle to maintain vision to a tragic conclusion. If the truth be known, it was more than likely a combination of factors that contributed to the loss of sight in these cases.

The story finally needed to be told concerning the culpability of the conventional medical community. Their hands are not clean in this matter. They do play a role in vision loss through these retinal injections based on their own admission and on the same admission that they "never play a role in the restoration of vision." This was exemplified by having told the patient on his or her very first encounter that "nothing can be done."

YOU MUST HAVE A PLAN

As you become more convinced that "something can be done," you will become emboldened to actually inform your doctor of your treatment plan as you see it. You are an adult. You are the patient. You are able to assess all your options. You then decide what your treatment options will be.

Once that decision is made, it can be amended at any time based on new information and new advisements from multiple sources, both professional and nonprofessional alike. This can only happen once you appreciate that your vision can be restored. It is my intention to take you there.

The Three-Step Program will improve your vision substantially in as short a period of time as three days. Once you are able to experience those vision gains, you will be ready to formulate a plan that will allow your input to be as important as anyone else's, including your eye doctor's.

It is now appropriate to discuss how such a plan may look. It is now time to explain the logic behind why one step should precede another. It may not be how your plan ultimately looks, but for discussion purposes, we will stick with the number three.

We have already introduced the concept of the Three-Step Program to return your sight. We also have mentioned that you can participate in an aggressive "Three-Day Program" to jump-start your vision restoration. Now let's discuss a "three-pronged decision plan" for any difficult decision when there are multiple options to consider.

Up until now, you have permitted your eye doctor to run the show. Now you run the show. You deserve to receive better vision immediately, and anything that prevents you from doing so should be dismissed from your plan.

Step 1

There is a problem with the game you are participating in that makes it biased against your best medical interests. The problem, which you will easily come to understand, is that you are consulting with an eye professional who is trained and paid to do injections into the retina of the eye. This is what the man does for a living. It could be argued, with a few minor exceptions, that it is the only thing he does for a living.

You come along with an eye disorder of wet ARMD for which there is no known medical cure. This doctor looks into the back of your eye and confirms that there is bleeding in the retina. After all, that is what wet ARMD is. At that point, the game is rigged and over. You will find that you will be scheduled for a retinal injection, if not that day then at his next available appointment.

By the way, one injection takes between fifteen and thirty seconds to complete. Also by the way, he is paid $2,000 to $3,000 to do that injection. Also by the way, I have had a patient describe a waiting room full of patients on injection day. There is no real limiting factor to a thirty-second procedure other than how many patients you can have lined up. Can you hear the "ka-ching" sound of a cash register?

Each of those patients will receive an injection. Each of the patients has wet ARMD. Each of the patients receives a medically appropriate procedure for a disease that has no cure, and nobody will ever question the care because it is considered medically appropriate.

To level the playing field that is tilted against you, it will be in your best medical interest to be evaluated by an eye professional that does not perform retinal injections. There are plenty of eye doctors who can do the eye examination and have no incentive to recommend for or against doing these injections.

Your own eye doctor will do, but an even better choice is to request an evaluation done by an optometrist and not an ophthalmologist. The reason I say this is that optometrists do not perform any procedures, so there is no bias toward doing retinal or any other injections. The other reason is that optometrists are excellent eye professionals in that their entire career has been spent monitoring patients both pre- and post-injection. Many of their patients may have actually been sent to the retinal specialist to be evaluated for a retinal injection.

This first examination only establishes a baseline. No matter what level of bleeding may be identified, this assessment is only meant to allow the optometrist to visually examine the extent of the bleed and to document it—only.

Step 2

At this point, you need to initiate the Three-Step Program either in-home or as a three-day in-office experience. You will have to let finances determine which approach you aggressively pursue. These modalities will be discussed in up-and-coming chapters in this book.

It is advantageous to you to compress the time frame to elicit the improvements possible in the three-day format. In-home modalities also exert a powerful restoration capability. Response times will be greater than three days, but they nonetheless will still occur. I have made this statement multiple times and will now repeat it: "Eighty-five to ninety percent of those patients who participate in the three-day treatment program will have a substantial improvement in their vision in three days."

If you elect to pursue in-home modalities, it would be beneficial to set your own time limit to achieve vision improvement. It may be your choice to construct a one-month or three-month program. It really does not matter which time frame you select. It only matters that you utilize the modalities I describe with enthusiasm and anticipation that there will be significant gains in your vision at the conclusion of your self-constructed program, and then move on to Step 3.

Step 3

It is now time to be reevaluated by your eye professional. It is extremely important that the same eye doctor that initially assessed you in Step 1 is the eye professional who reassessed you in Step 3. This doctor will remember your assessment both on visual inspection and notation made in your medical record.

It is important to note that we are discussing this plan as part of the presentation of wet ARMD. Because of that fact, the majority of patients are asking a common question, which is to be expected. "Do I have to get retinal injections from my ophthalmologist?" Many patients already have an appointment scheduled for their return visit to their eye doctor, and they are truly looking for a reason, any reason, to be able to at least put that appointment on hold.

I am most familiar with those patients confronted with this dilemma within the context of the three-day treatment program. In the many years I have been involved with this program, there have been very few patients who were recommended to keep their appointment with the retinal specialist. If you are anguishing over a similar situation of impending injection, your greatest opportunity to avoid that type of treatment lies within participating in the Three-Day Program.

I can only share with you my experience with the optometrist who works closely with me and those patients who participate in my in-office program. Her name is Dr. Lisa Bowen. She has her own thriving practice located close to my office.

About two and a half years ago, I met with her to ask her to become a part of our treatment programs. At that time, I told her that the three-day eye programs would be done in my office and that I really did need an eye professional to assess and evaluate those patients both at the beginning as well as the completion of the three days.

As I described the program, I went on to say:

The way this should work, Dr. Bowen, is that on Day 1, you and I will do assessments of these patients. After you and I have both completed those assessments, I am going to be working with these patients for three full days from nine o'clock in the morning until four o'clock in the afternoon.

On the third day, the very last thing I would like to do is send all the patients back to you so that you can reexamine them at that time.

Dr. Bowen looked a little confused. Quite frankly, she asked me why in the world these patients would need to come back to see her only three days after she initially evaluated them. It was at that point that I had to be honest and tell her, "By the way, Dr. Bowen, I fully expect that these patients will have tremendous improvements in three days. I would like you to assess them to verify that has, in fact, occurred."

At that point, Dr. Bowen rolled her eyes upward. She was looking at the sky as if to say, "Oh, my goodness. How is anybody going to have any improvement in three days?"

I should say that Dr. Bowen has become quite proud of the fact that she sees in these patients the tremendous turnarounds that we claim can and do occur with our help over the last two and a half years. Dr. Bowen is actually very excited to see these patients on Day 3 after having seen the level of pathology they exhibited just three days earlier.

I rely on her judgment implicitly, especially with making a decision as to whether or not these patients will require a retinal injection for bleeding that may be occurring in the back of their eye if they suffer from wet macular degeneration. The eye doctor you select will be more than happy to participate in advising you on how well you have done in the same endeavor.

Wet ARMD presents an interesting opportunity to become aware of the success of the Three-Step and Three-Day Programs. It has permitted many patients to discover the power behind integrative medicine approaches to severe medical problems and equally exposes some glaring weaknesses in conventional medicine. There are strengths and weaknesses in both. In the treatment of all retinal diseases, the conventional treatment approach fails miserably.

Let's continue with another representative of the category of retinal diseases.

GLAUCOMA

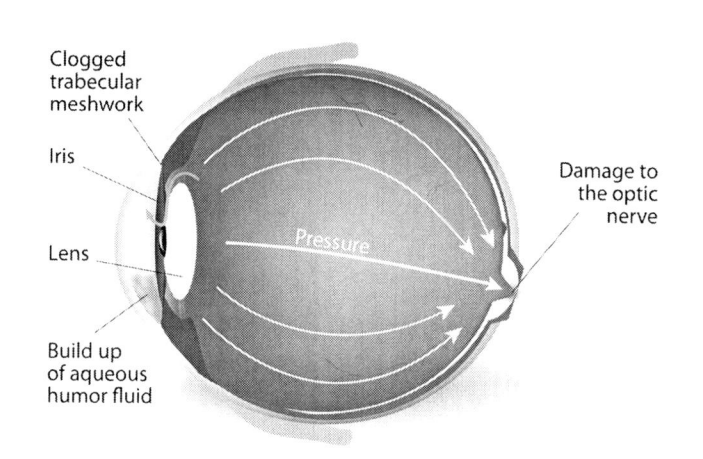

Glaucoma is a term that refers to a group of eye disorders that can cause damage to the retina as well as to the optic nerve. It is the second-leading cause of blindness in the United States behind macular degeneration, but it is the number-one cause of total blindness.

The normally functioning eye has two compartments. The anterior compartment is found in front of the lens and associated structures, and the posterior compartment lies behind the lens.

The posterior compartment is lined with a light-sensitive tissue known as the retina. The retina receives focused images that pass through the lens and then are transmitted to the brain through the optic nerve for recognition and interpretation.

The anterior compartment manufactures a constant amount of a clear fluid known as aqueous humor, which then circulates out of the anterior compartment through an intricate drainage system located in the corner of that compartment. It is an elaborate drainage system that allows the newly formed aqueous to flow out of that chamber. In so doing, the pressure created in the compartment is maintained at a normal and safe level as long as fluid is allowed to pass through the ultimate "drain plug" known as the trabecular meshwork.

If for any reason the drainage system is restricted or obstructed, the pressure in the chamber increases. That pressure increase is then transmitted to the posterior compartment which compresses the tiny capillary network of blood vessels which nourish the cells of the retina and, as a result, starve those very sensitive cells to that structure from a blood supply, leading to cell death.

It is common for glaucoma to develop with no warning whatsoever. The vision that is lost predominantly occurs in the patient's peripheral vision with central vision being unaffected. In a sense, the visual world closes in on the patient so insidiously that it goes unnoticed.

Unfortunately many patients with glaucoma seek medical attention after significant peripheral vision has already been lost. It is at that point he will be informed that "nothing can be done" to restore any vision that has already been lost and that all of the efforts from the eye professional will be directed to lowering intraocular pressures in an attempt to prevent further irrevocable eye damage and vision loss.

It is important to distinguish between two very different aspects of glaucoma. The first component of glaucoma is that it is a drainage disorder of the anterior eye. The second component of glaucoma is that it is a retinal disease that leads to vision loss.

Let me be clear from the onset that conventional medicine only attempts to intervene in correcting the drainage problem that has resulted in increased intraocular pressure (IOP). This is a vitally important treatment objective to lower IOP. There are numerous procedures available to the ophthalmologist to correct this drainage problem.

It should also be said that the Three-Step Program can and does lower intraocular pressure, but if these pressures cannot be lowered enough through non-invasive measures, everything in the arsenal of the eye doctor can and should be used. The pressures must be controlled at all costs, and a unique symbiotic relationship between conventional and alternative medical treatments should be successful in controlling this aspect of the disease.

The second component of glaucoma is that elevated intraocular pressure leads to the destruction of the retina. According to the medical profession, "nothing can be done" to restore any of the vision that has already been lost. I will avoid redundancy and simply say that you can restore your lost vision now through the use of the Three-Step Program.

A special mention is required concerning medications prescribed by your eye doctor in the form of eye drops that patients instill into the eyes on a daily basis. It is the policy of Dr. Edward Kondrot, a board certified ophthalmologist and originator of the three-day treatment program, never to direct any patient to discontinue those eye drops. The prescription medication should only be adjusted and/or discontinued by the eye doctor who prescribed them.

As your IOP decreases, your ophthalmologist will automatically lower the dosage of the drops. It is likely that when the IOP is lowered substantially, he will withdraw the medications completely. You should also continue consulting with another eye professional, who can provide you with a second opinion as they also follow your intraocular pressures.

Intraocular pressure is measured in millimeters of mercury, just as barometric pressure. There is actually no recognized normal intraocular pressure. These pressures are unique to each patient's own physiology, and it is quite common to find that eye professionals who know their patients will establish a "target" range of IOP that is specific to them alone.

It is quite obvious that intraocular pressures in excess of twenty millimeters of mercury are never considered acceptable. By the same token, there is one form of glaucoma that is often referred to as low-pressure glaucoma where damage can occur to the retina when intraocular pressures are extremely low. In either case, a target IOP will be established. Whatever means are necessary to bring patients into a safe and acceptable target range will become the standard for that particular patient.

With that being said, surgical procedures are possible to control intraocular pressures when all other measures have failed. In keeping with our philosophy, they should be considered a treatment option of last resort.

Once the pressure component of glaucoma has been managed successfully, and whether that management has consisted of conventional or alternative measures or combinations of both, the beginning of the vision restoration program we will be describing may commence. At that point, glaucoma becomes just another one of the many retinal diseases in which you can restore your vision with the Three-Step Program.

DIABETIC RETINOPATHY

Type 1 diabetes, known as insulin dependent, and type 2 diabetes, known as noninsulin dependent, are variations of a tumultuous disorder that does not spare any organ or body system. Even when blood-sugar levels are managed adequately, there are ultimately far-reaching consequences to a multiyear exposure of the mechanisms of this disease.

The unifying pathology responsible for the late manifestations of the disease is related to the cardiovascular sequelae that are all too frequently associated with diabetes. The diabetic is the first to have a heart attack, stroke, and kidney disease that frequently leads to dialysis and transplantation.

The diabetic is almost exclusively in that group of patients who develops wounds in the extremities, especially in the feet, that do not heal. The ultimate consequence is to develop a gangrenous extremity that requires amputation to spare the life of the patient.

Accumulation of plaque in the arteries is accelerated in the diabetic, but the plaque-deposition process is certainly not unique to diabetes. What is unique is that the most devastating consequence of diabetes is found in the microvasculature. These diseased microscopic arterial blood vessels are truly only found in diabetes. It is because of these deranged vascular structures that a normal blood supply to the tissues cannot be established to provide the nutrients and oxygen to the cells, so they cannot function normally.

It should come as no surprise that diabetes has serious implications with respect to the eye and to the retina in particular. It is said that it is impossible for a patient to suffer from diabetes for greater than thirty years without the retina being substantially involved. The conditions that result are together as a group known as diabetic retinopathy, which is associated with resultant loss of vision that can lead to total blindness.

A special mention should be made about the diabetic with retinal involvement in keeping with the Three-Step Program that is being discussed:

- Diabetic retinopathy is no different from any other retinal disease in how it responds to modalities that are used in the Three-Step Program. We continue to observe substantial improvement in vision in as short a period of time as three days.

- It was previously pointed out that diabetic retinopathy is a consequence to the pervasive manifestations of a diseased microvasculature. The diseased blood vessels leak fluid and bleed. As was pointed out during the discussion of wet ARMD, the same diseased retinal blood vessels also bleed. It is because of this that retinal specialists will recommend the same anti-VEGF injections to the patient with diabetic retinopathy that they did with the patients with wet ARMD.

The same plan that was suggested during that discussion is operational here. Go back and read it again. The three-pronged plan to avoid injections, in brief, is as follows:

1. Receive an evaluation from another eye doctor.

2. Complete a three-step and/or three-day treatment program.

3. Return to be reevaluated to see if your improvements permit you to avoid any invasive treatment at all.

ALL THE REST

We initially presented a lengthy list of the better-known retinal diseases in the previous chapter. As a group, they are all considered to have no possibility to be reversed in any way by conventional medical means.

The overarching theme we have continually introduced has been and continues to be that you can "restore your lost vision—now" through the Three-Step Program to regain your sight. That restoration can begin in as short of a period of time as three days.

In this chapter, we have pointed out that some of the retinal diseases earned the need of a special direct discussion. That need was earned not because of some remarkable sight-restoration contribution that just had to be brought to your attention. Instead, the need for a special discussion was to address potential harm that may await you by not making certain procedures a last resort instead of a first intention.

All remaining retinal diseases, as a rule, do not have special procedures that can lead to unintended consequences.

For that reason, we should bring this chapter to a conclusion on the same high note that continues to be intertwined and intermingled in the conversation from the beginning of this book. Let's proceed with the task of explaining the Three-Step Program to restore your sight.

CHAPTER 4

LET'S TAKE A STEP BACKWARD FOR A MOMENT

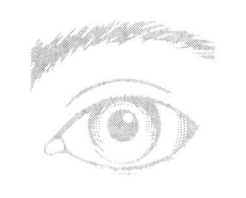

Before we delve into the unique Three-Step Program to regain your sight, it would serve us well to set the table appropriately by addressing a question that is repeatedly brought to my attention by a majority of patients who come under my care: How can such a program to restore vision be remotely possible and my eye doctor not even know about it? This troubling issue is actually an unavoidable one when it comes right down to it.

On its face, such a question makes good, logical sense. After all, your eye doctor has been trained to exhibit excellence and command in Western medicine. As a member of the American-educated contingent of medical practice, your doctor is understandably expected to be at the top of the heap.

With respect to these understandable assumptions, I wholeheartedly concur. The unfortunate reality, however, is that your doctor can only master that which is presented to him. On those medical matters, he is the expert and is well deserving of our admiration and respect.

The issue then becomes what ends up being taught to our doctors that results in what will be able to be mastered? This is where our medical professionals are at an extreme disadvantage. The academic powers that be have predetermined that 97 percent of what will be taught to our doctors is already etched in granite. The evaluation of that medical slate has evolved for more than a hundred years.

Early on in this struggle, many approaches to treating human diseases were just discarded. One such approach that was well rooted in accepted medical practice at that time was that of homeopathy, which was introduced in 1796 by Samuel Hahnemann. Hahnemann Medical College was the first medical school in the United States and was established in 1848. Homeopathy and many other fields of medical endeavor were all vanquished by the 1920s.

To attest to the legacy of homeopathy, the Food and Drug Administration continues to control all prescription forms of homeopathic remedies with the same vigor as it exerts to control and monitor the use of pharmaceutical drugs.

By the beginning of the 1900s, homeopathy was thrown out, and drugs were welcomed in. The bulk of that medical school curriculum slate was set in granite, never to be looked back to again. By today's point in the evolutionary process of medical education, you cannot receive a coherent answer by any medical graduate if you ask him what homeopathy even is.

From the moment organized medicine made the decision that drugs and surgery were to be pronounced supreme, the firewall to insulate against all who should attempt to gain entrance and alter that determination must do so through "evidence-based medicine" (EBM).

EBM is the code word that on the surface sounds so legitimate. Below the surface, it is plagued with at least the potential to be misused and truly abused. The medical agenda has been determined. Ninety-seven percent of what will be taught is already established medical dogma. What remains, the approximately 3 percent that is left over, will gain final acceptance through medical studies alone.

It is in this way that the door is nailed shut for innovation and new approaches to treat human disease. It is the primary reason your doctor does not know and is not going to know about a three-step or twelve-step or hundred-step program to correct any form of human dysfunction.

For that reason, an explanation is in order. Since the use of drugs was elected to be the standard bearer for organized Western medicine and the US Food and Drug Administration (FDA) as the agency to be the gatekeeper for that standard, the stage has been set for what can be elevated to occupy the remaining 3 percent of the total of medical dogma.

It had been the pharmaceutical industry that readily recognized the opening, no matter how small, and realized it is economically to their advantage to aggressively participate in the medical-study process to have a chance to obtain a hold of the brass ring of medicine—an FDA-approved drug—that comes with exclusivity and a patent to maintain that exclusivity for a minimum of twenty years after the drug has been invented.

It is estimated that it will take at least eight years of study after inventing the drug to accumulate enough data to take that drug past the US Food and Drug Administration scrutiny to determine that it is both safe and effective.

We could have an extensive discussion about the issue of safety and effectiveness, but that subject is outside the scope of our current discussion, which is to explain why your doctor has such a terrible time understanding how there can even be something called a Three-Step Program to regain your sight.

On matters of safety, one only needs to turn to an evening of commercial television for the next drug advertisement to appear. During the last fifteen seconds of the ad, someone begins talking at about a hundred-mile-per-hour pace to let you know it is possible for you to experience that one of your legs might fall off, an eye could pop out of your head, and, by the way, you could drop over dead from taking this drug. So much for the safe and effective for now—I will let you form your own decision about that.

The point I want to make is this. A new report published by the Tufts Center for the Study of Drug Development published in November 2014 puts the cost of developing a new drug that gains market approval at $2.6 billion. This is a 145 percent increase corrected for inflation over the estimate made by the same center in 2003. I will let you calculate what that may mean for the cost of bringing a drug to market today.

The components of a study that determine the cost are things like randomized, placebo controlled, double blind, crossover, and others. In round numbers, each word actually employed by those funding the study appears to be going at a rate of about $500 million per word.

Besides the unbelievable amount of money that is required to demonstrate the validity that a drug is "safe and effective," another issue concerning medical studies has created a great deal of cynicism among many of my colleagues, including myself. There appear to be many doctors who have come to realize that you can construct a study to come up with the result you are looking for to begin with. It is for this reason that we in the profession have come to pick and choose the studies that support our own personal viewpoint and reject those that do not.

This little-understood reality by the lay public is a fair personal admission to reveal during the current discussion. If there is a way for closely held medical beliefs to be turned upside down, a medical study or so-called evidence-based medicine will be sure to do it.

I wonder how the following list of universally held medical truths would do up against the close scrutiny of a medical study:

- An apple a day will keep the doctor away.

- Do everything in moderation.

- Take plenty of vitamin D daily.
- Sleep at least eight hours per night.

Do not put it past medical science to construct a study to take on any one of the previously accepted truths about good health. That study is waiting just around the corner.

This conversation started because of the frequent questions asked by patients regarding the Three-Step Program. It is certainly legitimate to ask of something out there, "Is that good? Why doesn't my doctor know about it?" What I believe should become obvious is not only does he not know about it, but he will not know about it any time in the near future either.

As a final point to close that discussion completely, I should add that if he should ever entertain the idea that such a program does exist, he would refuse to investigate it any further because it would not be in his financial best interests to do so.

To emphasize this point, allow me to share with you a personal story. It involves a cardiologist friend of mine who has been coming to my office every other week for the last fifteen years. He has been extremely important to my practice because he has provided my patients with an extremely detailed and sophisticated cardiovascular assessment that I have believed is vital in correcting cardiovascular disease.

For this assessment, the blood work that I consider as standard for all patients consists of eighteen specific blood tests to objectively quantify blood markers that influence cardiovascular risk.

Let's be clear. I did not invent these eighteen blood tests. Medical science determined their value and importance. They then introduced those eighteen blood markers into the medical literature. The moment the medical literature described each and every one of them, all medical doctors read those descriptions. Being the good doctors they are, they made them part of their medical acumen. If you ask any doctor about any one of the eighteen markers, they will give you fifteen to twenty minutes of "off-the-cuff" explanation to explain how potentially harmful each of them could be.

At this point, it becomes a little embarrassing. You see, even knowing the potential harm associated with each of the markers individually, much less collectively, the doctors do not and will not order seventeen of the eighteen blood tests as part of the workup for their patients.

Even though that may seem odd, I will reveal to you that as it stands today, medical science has no "medicine" to correct those seventeen markers. By "medicine," I want to specify that there is no drug to correct the marker should it be elevated. In a way, you had better thank your lucky stars that the drug companies never find a "medicine" to correct these markers. As I usually like to say, "You will need to have a wheelbarrow to get out of your doctor's office with all the drug samples that will be heaped upon you."

Let's return to my cardiologist. After fifteen years of evaluating my patients from his perspective as a specialist with lab work that I have selected and that appear on their individual results that are indirectly in front of him, surely he observed how the markers were corrected and trended to arrive into a normal range.

Here comes the punch line. With all the improvements in those eighteen markers that he had to observe, and for sure understanding there was no drug from the pharmaceutical industry that had even the possibility of doing the same, you would think he would have at least asked me what I did to make those changes happen. There has been fifteen years of dead silence. There has been nothing. There has not been even the slightest bit of inquisitiveness.

Truth be told, I harbor no ill will toward my very competent cardiologist colleague. The fact that our relationship ever started to begin with was his willingness to provide his expertise when other cardiologists did not even want to admit they knew me. Well, they may not have known me, but they certainly knew of me. They did not want to have anything to do with me and whatever my methods were.

My cardiologist, in my opinion, never asked me about the eighteen markers because it was not in his best financial interest to do so. Any specialist lives and dies by the referral. You as a patient do not just go to a cardiologist, gastroenterologist, or any -ologist. You are referred to a specialist by your primary-care physician (PCP).

If you as a specialist want to keep those referrals coming, do not do anything to rock the boat. Do not be innovative. Do not move into territory that may confuse the referral source. Do not start ordering blood tests that may allow your referral source to call your actions into question. If you do so, it will not be too long before those referral sources will dry up. When they dry up, your practice will go belly up.

The medical profession does not like it when you rock the boat. You should not expect your eye doctor to know about the Three-Day Program. You will have to take it upon yourself to explore it and ultimately decide to participate in it or not. After all, it is your vision and not your eye doctor's vision that is deteriorating. That in itself is reason enough to learn more.

THE ONLY STUDY THAT MATTERS: RESULTS

Having at least exposed the potential for bias that can be reflected in the results of a medical study, and detailing the undeniable expense required to bring a new drug to the market ($2.6 billion), it should be clear that only the "big boys" receive an opportunity to participate in the medical treatment game.

There has been remarkable work done by teams of investigators in the past. Their work is exemplary. Their methods are flawless. The ultimate conclusions that were drawn both deserved and became the bedrock of traditional medicine.

We have also been made aware of those investigators who have been dishonest and lacked the integrity required to conduct an unbiased study. Those investigators yielded to the pressures of their institutions to publish research papers and the temptation of the pharmaceutical industry's financial incentives to have the study conclude what the drug company required it to conclude to keep their product within the good graces of the FDA.

Those farcical studies have usually been kept nice and tidy. The only injured party turns out to be the public who places its trust in the process as well as the federal agencies that have been created to protect it.

There is no realistic way alternative medicine can compete with the pharmaceutical complex in the formation of a new treatment no matter how miraculous that treatment may be. The process by its very design is meant to dismiss all commerce, no matter what their intention, to have a seat at the table. You need to have $2.6 billion to even sit at the table if you want to be taken seriously.

There is a way, however, to not just take a seat but to participate in an effective and adequate assessment of a new and innovative treatment that can go toe-to-toe with the drug complex and assure the public it meets the requirements of being both safe and effective. The term that most adequately describes this type of study can be summed up in one word: results.

Is the Program Safe?

Drug companies are at an unbelievable disadvantage of their own creation. You see, they have instructed their research and development divisions to create a "synthetic" molecule to perform a specific task. The task may, and does, continually change. It may be, for instance, to lower blood pressure, prevent seizures, or lower blood-sugar levels. The list of the tasks is endless.

The one thing that remains the same for all drug companies, however, is that the substance must be synthetic. It has to be a molecule that they and only they have created in the lab. If the substance resembles any naturally occurring molecule at all, they lose. What is lost turns out to be the holy grail of all drug companies, which is the patent to produce the drug.

To risk $2.6 billion on a project, a drug must be a one-of-a-kind "franken" molecule that does not exist in nature. If the substance cannot meet these unique criteria, there is no patent or exclusivity to guarantee a return on investment. That return exponentially exceeds the $2.6 billion it costs the drug company initially that will keep their company and their investors quite content as long as the medical doctors will now hopefully prescribe the drug to their patients.

I started this discussion about return on investment by mentioning that the drug company is at a distinct disadvantage with their new product. Remember, this new drug is a synthetic, one-of-a-kind, foreign substance "franken" molecule. As a result of this inescapable fact, you cannot introduce such a substance into the human body without provoking unintended consequences.

If the instruction given to the research and development division was, for example, to lower a person's blood pressure, it will be my guess that the drug will do that with varying degrees of effectiveness. The problem will be that the new substance will interact with every other tissue in the body and lead to unwanted, undesirable, and yes, even lethal consequences.

We medical doctors have a very thick book that sits on our desk known as the PDR (*Physician's Desk Reference*). During each drug study, prior to receiving approval, any side effect experienced by even one patient must be documented and will appear in the PDR. Some of these complications are minor. Many are not. The fact that you can obtain a patent to make a medicine that meets the FDA standard of being "safe" yet has so much potential for harm is inconceivable to me.

It should be obvious that this matter will not be resolved here. I felt it important only to explain the advantage of an alternative approach where there are minimal to no safety issues concerning your participation in the Three-

Step Program. The point is we use no drugs. We do not even use any natural substance that acts like a drug. There are no safety issues to consider. You cannot be harmed in any way by your participation in the program.

This new approach allows me to explain the remaining criteria that must always be considered in assessing a medical therapy. Is it effective?

Is the Program Effective?

Once the matter of safety has been adequately explained and addressed, the only other aspect of any medical therapy should go directly to the issue of whether the therapy is effective.

In a medical study run by a drug company, effectiveness requires a number of steps. The first is that the individuals participating in the study are selected randomly. That means that for those who have been selected to participate, half of the patients actually receive the drug. The other half does not. Instead, that half receives a placebo or sugar tablet that looks the same as the real drug but has no potential to alter biological activity. No one knows whether they are in the group that is actually receiving the drug or not.

In our program, there is no randomization. All participants receive all the therapy all the time. There are no placebos used. Everyone who has a serious retinal disease will be given the opportunity to obtain the full benefit of the Three-Step Program. The components of "double blind" and "crossover" are not even operational in our program because of the full participation of all patients in all aspects of the program, both at the office facility and at home.

When all is said and done, there is no need for complicated mathematical algorithms to assess the effectiveness of the Three-Step Program. We are extremely proud of our results. We do not know of any other program with a track record even remotely resembling our own and that has been established in its present form for more than ten years.

The standards for assessing the results of our program are simply this: At the beginning of the program, the patients are assessed. Three days of aggressive nondrug and nonsurgical modalities are administered. At the conclusion, patients are reassessed using the same objective parameters utilized at the start of the program.

When all is said and done, "Eighty-five to ninety percent of all those patients that have participated in the program have demonstrated a substantial improvement in their vision in three days."

Here are the actual results experienced by the patients who completed the program over a three-year period and the list of the diagnoses they presented with at the time of their participation in the program.

RESULTS

Here is a list of patients treated and their results after the Three-Day Program.

Improvement of *acuity* is listed in either lines (five letters in a line) or letters better.

Improvement of *contrast* is listed in the number of additional letters read.

Improvement of *visual fields* is listed as follows:

    MINIMAL: 0 to 5 degrees expansion of the visual field

    MODERATE: 5 to 10 degrees

    MARKED: greater than 10 degrees

ARMD Dry – 70 patients
Glaucoma – 29 Patients
ARMD wet – 20 patients

Macular Hole, Macular Wrinkling, Pucker – 9 patients

Stargardts – 3 patients

Cataracts – 6 patients

Ischemic Optic Nerve Disease – 4 patients

Retinitis Pigmentosa – 4 patients

Diabetic Retinopathy – 3 patients

Histoplasmosis Scarring – 3 patients

Cone Dystrophy – 1 patient

RESULTS OF ALL 152 PATIENTS, OR 290 EYES TREATED

ACUITY IMPROVEMENT

2 lines (10 letters) or better: 43 eyes / 15%

1 line (5 letters) or better: 158 eyes / 54%

1 to 4 letters better: 66 eyes / 23%

No change: 23 eyes / 8%

CONTRAST IMPROVEMENT

5 or more letters better: 104 eyes / 36%

1 to 4 letters better: 151 / 52%

No change: 35 eyes / 12%

VISUAL FIELD EXPANSION

Marked: 165 eyes / 57%

Moderate: 75 eyes / 26%

Minimal: 19 eyes / 6%

No change: 31 eyes / 11%

ARMD DRY

70 patients, 140 eyes
Average improvement of acuity: 5.5 letters
Average improvement of contrast: 3.8 letters

ACUITY IMPROVEMENT

2 lines or greater: 22 eyes
1 to 2 lines: 53 eyes
Less than one line: 50 eyes
No change: 15 eyes

CONTRAST IMPROVEMENT

Greater than 6 letters: 35 eyes
3 to 5 letters: 38 eyes
1 to 2 letters: 54 eyes
No change: 13 eyes

VISUAL FIELD EXPANSION

Marked: 76 eyes
Moderate: 41 eyes
No change or minimal: 23 eyes

GLAUCOMA

29 patients, 58 eyes
Average change in acuity: 6 letters
Average change in contrast: 3.6 letters
Average drop in pressure: 4.8 mm HG

ACUITY IMPROVEMENT

2 lines or greater: 10 eyes

1 to 2 lines: 26 eyes
Less than one line: 16 eyes
No change: 6 eyes

CONTRAST IMPROVEMENT

Greater than 6 letters: 17 eyes
3 to 5 letters: 14 eyes
1 to 2 letters: 17 eyes
No change: 10 eyes

VISUAL FIELD EXPANSION

Marked: 37 eyes
Moderate: 14 eyes
No change or minimal: 7 eyes

PRESSURE LOWERING

Greater than 5 mm Hg lowering: 13 eyes
1 to 5 mm Hg lowering: 27 eyes
*No change: 11 eyes
*Increase in pressure: 7 eyes
*The majority of these patients stopped their eye drops, so pressure elevation or lack of response could be due to stopping medication.

ARMD WET

20 patients, 40 eyes
Average improvement of acuity: 6.4 letters
Average improvement of contrast: 5.0 letters

ACUITY IMPROVEMENT

2 lines or greater: 8 eyes

1 to 2 lines: 11 eyes
Less than one line: 20 eyes
No change: 1 eye

CONTRAST IMPROVEMENT

Greater than 6 letters: 11 eyes
3 to 5 letters: 9 eyes
1 to 2 letters: 13 eyes
No change: 7 eyes

VISUAL FIELD EXPANSION

Marked: 26 eyes
Moderate: 8 eyes
No change or minimal: 6 eyes

STARGARDTS

3 patients, 6 eyes

ACUITY IMPROVEMENT

Average acuity: 6.6 improvement
Range: 2 to 13 letters improvement

CONTRAST IMPROVEMENT

Average contrast: 3.67 improvement
Range: 0 to 10 letters

VISUAL FIELD

All had a marked improvement.

RETINITIS PIGMENTOSA, RP

4 patients, 8 eyes

ACUITY IMPROVEMENT
Average acuity: 15.3 letters better
Range: 0 to 68 letters

CONTRAST IMPROVEMENT
Average contrast: 3.1 letters better
Range: 0 to 8 letters

VISUAL FIELD EXPANSION
Marked expansion: 4 eyes
Moderate expansion: 2 eyes
Able to see color previously unable: 1 eye
No change: 1 eye

MACULAR HOLE, MACULAR WRINKLING, MACULAR PUCKER, ETC.

9 patients, 10 eyes

ACUITY IMPROVEMENT
Average acuity change: 4.3 letters better
Range: 0 to 11 letters

CONTRAST IMPROVEMENT
Average contrast: 2.5 letters better
Range: 0 to 8 letters

VISUAL FIELD EXPANSION
Marked: 3 eyes

Moderate: 4 eyes
Minimal: 3 eyes

CATARACTS

6 patients, 10 eyes

ACUITY IMPROVEMENT
Average acuity change: 5.75 letters better
Range: 0 to 16 letters

CONTRAST IMPROVEMENT
Average contrast 2.3 letters better
Range: 0 to 6 letters

VISUAL FIELD EXPANSION
Marked: 7 eyes
Moderate: 1 eye
None to slight: 2 eyes

ISCHEMIC OPTIC NEUROPATHY

4 patients, 6 eyes

ACUITY IMPROVEMENT
Average acuity: 5.75 letters
Range: 0 to 15 letters

CONTRAST IMPROVEMENT
Average change in contrast: 3.75 letters
Range: 0 to 6 letters

VISUAL FIELD EXPANSION

Marked: 3 eyes

Moderate: 3 eyes

DIABETIC RETINOPATHY

3 patients, 6 eyes

ACUITY IMPROVEMENT

Average acuity: 7.8 letters

Range: 3 to 17 letters

CONTRAST IMPROVEMENT

Average contrast: 5.5 letters

Range: 2 to 11 letters

VISUAL FIELD EXPANSION

Marked: 4 eyes

Moderate: 2 eyes

HISTOPLASMOSIS RETINAL SCARRING

3 patients, 4 eyes

ACUITY IMPROVEMENT

Average acuity: 4 letters

Range: 2 to 11 letters

CONTRAST IMPROVEMENT

Average contrast: 7.3 letters

Range: 3 to 12 letters

VISUAL FIELD EXPANSION
Marked in all eyes, 2 had reduction in blind spots

CONE DYSTROPHY

1 patient, 2 eyes

ACUITY IMPROVEMENT
Average acuity: 5 letters
Range: 4 to 6 letters

CONTRAST IMPROVEMENT
Average Contrast: 1 letter
Range: 0 to 2 letters

VISUAL FIELD
Moderate both eyes

If It Is Going to Happen, It Will Have to Be Alternative

It should be abundantly clear by now that the agenda is set in the conventional-medical arena. It is not within the sphere of credibility of eye doctors that what is considered to be "dead" retinal tissue can ever be brought back to any level of functioning once again.

They do lament that "nothing can be done," but if you suffer from a retinal disease, the empathy you receive from your doctor is but a small consolation to what the impending doom of your disease has been forecasted to do, which is to either gradually or rapidly progress. It should also be abundantly clear that if any major advancement is to be possible in reversing retinal disease, it will need to come from alternative medicine and not conventional.

There is no formal alternative training for doctors who wish to pursue alternative medicine as a model for their practice. To be at least moderately conciliatory concerning our conventional doctors, there is so much that needs to be learned during the medical education of our doctors. There really is not any time left to include alternatives to conventional medicine.

Of the thousands of diseases that are studied by our current medical students, each disease is addressed individually. That means each disease has its own unique cause or causes. Each has its own multitude of signs and symptoms that allow it to be clinically differentiated from one another. Each has a myriad of laboratory tests, radiographic studies, and other specific tests to assist in accurately making the correct diagnosis.

When all that has been done effectively and the treatments are to be considered, usually multiple drugs can be selected, each of which has its own unique profile and potential for risk and drug reactions. These reactions are only unique to each particular patient and are based on his or her own personal history and reactivity with any other medication that he or she may already be taking.

Let's be laudatory for a moment. Your doctor is brilliant. He had to be in order to learn all that was required of him to graduate from medical school and then to do it all over again when his three-year residency program had finally concluded.

This encapsulation of a medical education is why I immediately bestow my utmost respect to all my colleagues and medical collaborators. We all share this common experience and have emerged to service the medical needs of our individual communities. At this point, the success of the doctor will be determined by a plethora of personality attributes and human frailties by which a final decision will be rendered. That decision will be made by the recipient of that accumulated skill set—the patient himself.

CHAPTER 4: LET'S TAKE A STEP BACKWARD FOR A MOMENT

As much as I admire my fellow clinicians for the accomplishments of surviving a medical education, I would be remiss if I did not expose two of the most disturbing and glaring negative attributes that, although not universal, are nonetheless pervasive in conventional medicine.

In the one instance, a tragic personality flaw appears to be given an opportunity to be expressed, and that opportunity is rarely ignored. In the second instance, the delusion is that conventional medical management has no equal and that, in fact, is far superior to any other form of medical intervention. They truly believe that those who pursue such alternative medical approaches do so as a result of ignorance and not enlightenment.

As for the first point, the most repeated criticism that patients relate to me with respect to their encounters with their own doctors from conventional medicine is the extreme arrogance displayed by the doctors in responding to their inquiries regarding alternative options.

Whatever question has been asked by the patient regarding alternative modalities, the direct verbal or indirect nonverbal response is a resounding, "You can't be serious" or "You must be kidding" retort that rapidly produces the desired behavior that the doctor is really attempting to provoke. That, of course, is for the patient to acquiesce, become silent, and allow the atmosphere in the office to return back to the comfort level of the doctor once again.

Unbeknownst to the doctor, however, an entirely different set of behaviors has been put in play. The patient, who was initially seeking to become a partner with the doctor in medical matters, now understands that no such partnership is possible, and if he desires to be treated according to his wishes, he will obviously require another doctor in future plans.

Let me reveal what your doctor could not. In doing so, it might soften the blow that you either had to endure or have yet to experience. The fact of the matter is whatever question was asked, your very brilliant and highly trained doctor realized almost immediately that he did not have a clue how to answer your question.

This professional who is so intelligent, precise, and instructive in all medical matters has just been fed a question that reduced an inquiry to a medical version of an old TV show entitled *Let's Stump the Band*. When you ask them, "What about my diet?" he realizes he has no medical-school cure on diet to fall back on. Forget about a course on diet. Your doctor has not had more than a thirty-minute lecture on diet. Obviously, you "stumped the band."

If you ask, "What about a vitamin?" there is no information up there in the gray or white matter that allows him to respond with the factual information you assumed he had to advise you about vitamins. As a result, you "stumped the band."

Even though the questions are simple ones, whenever the vast majority of physicians are confronted with them, they immediately feel so inadequate about being unable to answer them they respond with arrogant snippets in order to shield their own inadequacy on the subject.

I hope that my meager attempt to explain an embarrassing indiscretion that both you and your doctor may have experienced should not diminish how you feel about your doctor. He still is the intelligent individual that you always thought he was but in conventional matters alone.

If you are earnestly seeking usable information about an alternative therapy, ask an alternative doctor. The doctor you approach could be a chiropractor, naturopath, or homeopath. In each case, you will not trigger a personality flaw by merely seeking information.

I would urge you to consider seeking that advice from another MD or DO (osteopath) who practices integrative or alternative medicine. As a member of the medical profession with a medical education similar to your current doctor, he will immediately be able to explain the void in conventional medical education but, even more importantly, why pursuing alternative therapies will bring a host of possibilities to correct your medical condition that does not currently exist in established Western medicine.

As for the second negative attribute, it is universally understood by all doctors that conventional medical management has no equal in correcting disease and is far superior to any other form of medical intervention that may be offered by others now or in the future.

That is one big gulp for anyone to even actually think, let alone boldly verbalize, with a straight face. Your doctor figures if there was anything you claim may be possible to help you with your medical challenge, he, as a medical doctor, would have to at least have heard about it.

With your question presented and after quickly inventorying what he was taught and realizing that no such treatment, therapy, or modality has been discussed in his entire medical education, he can dismiss that treatment summarily as having no value whatsoever. This type of verbal discourse happens daily in the world of the medical doctor. As to whether you accept his response as valid or accurate usually says more about you rather than him.

The doctor's problem is that he lacks information and has already decided he will not be looking for any additional information on the subject anytime soon. You, on the other hand, suffer from a medical problem that he has not been able to correct. If you do not pursue obtaining additional information, your condition remains static, and your complaint, no matter how minor, will linger forever.

CHAPTER 5

THE PLEDGE AND THE PLAN

FIRST – THE PLEDGE
YOU WILL BE SUCCESSFUL WITH KISS

During my teaching career, my third-grade class of long ago instilled in me a rule that I never violate either with a class or with a patient. That cornerstone of education is well reconciled but rarely followed. You see, you can teach any of the most scientifically difficult and complex concepts if you just Keep It Simple, Stupid (KISS).

At the conclusion of any teaching session, a blank stare on the face of the audience or the patient means that the only person in the room who actually is stupid is the teacher himself for not simplifying the content of the discussion enough. If you seek mastery by your student, simplify your explanation, and you will see the light bulb glow in the eyes of your student. That signifies "Don't worry; I've got it."

There is a soothing reality worthwhile in coming across to your patient and in keeping with the KISS approach. That is that there is something alluring and comfort provoking about the number "three." If you want your patient to be willing to hang in there without prematurely bailing out on you, be sure you are clear from the beginning that there will not be a lengthy amount of time required to hear the message the physician (or teacher) wishes to deliver.

To prove that point, I do not think you would be reading this book if it were subtitled "The Twenty-Step Program to Regain Your Sight." Human nature suggests you would more than likely have said to yourself, "I don't have time to do twenty steps of anything," and moved on. The number three begs to be embraced. It is comfortable. It is doable.

In keeping with the KISS approach to simplify complex material and to make it more understandable, this chapter will present a Three-Step Program to restore your lost vision in its conceptual form. For this reason, this is the most important single chapter in the entire book.

As will be revealed in the next section, the power of the Three-Step Program is universal. Once you have laid down these three steps in your mind and committed them to memory, you will have discovered the starting point to correct not only your eye disease but also most of the other diseases of aging. It will become apparent later on as to what the specific modalities will be to accomplish the Three-Step Program. For now, keep your focus on the number three, which can be easily handled without being overwhelming.

The explanation of each of the steps will make such logical sense that you will not become bogged down by the minutia of medical complexity because the foundation of what you are about to learn can and will always be reduced to the number three. We will start simple and keep it simple. We will not lose you on the way to restoring your lost vision now.

SECOND – THE PLAN
THE POWER OF THE PLAN

I would now like to confide in you a secret. Actually, it is not a secret. Instead, it is the foundation of alternative medicine. It also turns out to be the reason alternative medicine can reverse disease when all of conventional medicine has failed.

I am consulted by numerous patients, and you can imagine that the range of medical problems presented to me is enormous. There are no two patients alike, even if two individuals have been diagnosed with the same disease. What remains as the main stumbling block with conventional treatment is that the entire focus is directed to fighting a disease when, in fact, all efforts must be directed to the restoration of health.

You cannot win if you are in a fight with a disease. The forces of the disease process are too overpowering to permit it to be defeated in combat when you realize that the drugs used in your medical management by your doctor are by their very design meant to alleviate symptoms and not to conquer disease. As you can see, you were never going to fight your disease anyway.

Supplying that cold dose of reality suggests that even the drug companies themselves realize you cannot beat a disease into submission. At best, it is possible to alleviate the symptoms of a disease to allow it to be tolerated better, but that disease will be operational and symptom provoking forever. Your only option, as you may have determined, will be to continue the medication, appreciate the symptom relief, and accept that the disease and you are inseparable forever.

Diseases only become reversible when the arsenals raised to correct them no longer attempt to beat the disease but to instead cultivate health. This paradigm shift is universally potent. It is the banner hoisted by the alternative and integrative medical complex and clearly delineates the sharp distinction between the two competing medical approaches.

The possibilities become endless when the mind-set shift occurs. You can reverse disease. You can nurture so-called "dead tissue" back to function again because it was never really dead to begin with. It was only assumed to be dead and irreversible because it was being treated as a disease and not as the absence of health. Once you begin to provide the components of health, you can and will have the possibility of fully functioning tissue once again.

The components to reestablish health are not complex. To the contrary, they are quite simple. The components are also not numerous. They are minimal. The starting point, as has been alluded to from the beginning point of this book, has been clearly announced. There are three steps required to be followed to restore function to diseased and dysfunctional tissue. Let me be clear that this plan is universally potent. I follow it with all patients in all diseases. It is particularly powerful when applied to diseases of the eye.

As a precaution, it should be clearly stated that in all cases currently being managed by your conventional medical doctor and for which you have been prescribed medication, nothing should change initially. You should continue to take any medication you are taking. No patient is ever directed or permitted to abruptly terminate the use of any medicine prescribed by their current doctors.

What you can more than likely expect to happen is that as you progress and improve, both you and your doctor will recognize that you do not require the use of the medication. The two of you together can decide that the drug is not required any longer. This important consideration is most critical, for instance, in glaucoma where intraocular pressure must be maintained in a safe range to protect against further vision loss.

With this important precaution clearly addressed, it is time to examine the plan, the Three-Step Program to regain your sight.

STEP 1: CORRECT ALL DEFICIENCIES

The discussion we are about to have cannot happen with your conventionally trained doctor. His education is devoid of any of the components necessary to intelligently address this monumentally important aspect in restoring health. On the other hand, most—if not all—clinicians in the alternative domain can be of great help and assistance by sharing their insight and can intelligently complement this discussion.

All human tissue possesses highly intricate metabolic activity that allows that tissue to function in a healthy manner. The core component demonstrated in any cell remains the same in all tissue no matter the organ or body system involved. Those core elements are

- to supply the cell with a source of energy in the form of a carbohydrate or fat; and

- to allow the mitochondria—the energy powerhouse of a cell—to convert the food source of energy into a chemical form of energy known as ATP (adenosine triphosphate).

Once ATP is available, the cell is permitted to carry out its specific function, which makes it unique. In the heart, ATP results in a muscle rhythmically contracting to move blood through the blood vessels. In the liver, ATP production allows liver cells to detoxify harmful substances found in the blood. In the eye, focused light that excites nervous tissue can convey an image to the brain where it can be interpreted as sight. A list of different body tissues results in the unique function of that body system, and all systems working in harmony with one another lead to establishing health.

Most of us do not have a problem supplying the adequate food source so that the body can produce energy in the form of ATP. There is another level of nutrients we do not supply in adequate amounts, and it is the lack of this group of nutrients that causes us trouble. A food source alone supplies the raw ingredients for a cell to produce energy, but there is a multitude of vitamins and minerals required to allow a cell to carry out specific functions in an optimal way.

A person's diet has evolved over a lifetime. Our tastes have resulted in a preferential selection of foods that we enjoy. The economics of a family also help in shaping what the diet of the family will be. The point that needs to be made is that each of us has accrued a host of nutritional deficiencies as a result of our diet. As a result of these deficiencies, there is always a metabolic pathway that is dramatically affected when even one nutrient is lacking, let alone when multiple nutrients have been absent over the course of a lifetime.

In our youth, there is great latitude in the tissues for compensating for nutritional deficiencies. This physiological reality has been collectively referred to as "the immortality of youth." During this time in our lives, if we lack a nutrient or a group of nutrients, our bodies have the capability of doing a metabolic workaround that allows the body to compensate for the deficiency and carry on the body process without any noticeable effect.

As we age, this ability to compensate for deficiency through metabolic "workarounds" is gradually but profoundly lost. For this reason, macular degeneration is not a disease of our twenty-year-olds. Glaucoma, with only rare exception, is absent in the thirty-year-old population. Diabetic retinopathy is only rarely seen in the young.

The aforementioned eye disorders are found predominantly in those individuals of advancing age. This undeniable fact is a direct result of a lifetime's worth of nutrient deficiencies finally manifesting in the tissues, causing them to not function properly and even furthering dysfunction.

It is unfortunate but accurate that the sum total of your body's deficiencies, although concealed under the surface, will come to the surface eventually. Individuals who do not correct this disturbance will pay the price for those deficiencies eventually.

The eye diseases of our advanced years were preventable. Not having dealt with their inevitability at an earlier period of our life is what has resulted in the age-related diseases we confront today. The point of emphasis, however, is that it is not too late to correct those deficiencies and reverse the conditions that have resulted from them.

YOU CAN REVERSE YOUR EYE DISEASE BY CORRECTING YOUR DEFICIENCIES

Your eye tissue is not dead. It is just unable to function correctly because nutrients required for that functioning have been missing from your diet for, in many cases, a lifetime. Only when these nutrients are finally provided will the journey back to health commence.

A geological analogy of an equivalent situation will serve us well at this time. There are places on this planet that have endured unimaginable hardship by enormous forces of nature that have changed the productivity of a large swath of a region from self-sustaining to a region of desolation. There are agricultural regions in the United States that, as we speak, have gone from abundant to disastrous.

By either divine intervention or man-made manipulation, the region can be restored to fully functional and self-sustaining once again. The point is no matter how bad it may have become in that area of the country, it was possible to revive it when the proper nutrients and water arrived.

The eye and its associated structures have become ground zero for the human equivalent of an agricultural drought. If it can be effectively provided with the nutrients that are lacking, it can function again. There is no drug that can reverse the havoc created by the absence of nutrients that have accrued over a lifetime.

Simply put, there is nothing synthetic that could take the place of the naturally derived substances of life. We will explore the options available to accomplish the task in the most expeditious manner possible. It is an odd twist of reality, however, that the correction of your deficiencies will not be compensated for by food alone.

As much as it makes intuitive good sense to improve your diet to combat a lack of nutrients, the reality is that you cannot ever achieve your intended goals by diet alone. At this point, the nutritional deficiencies are so great that extraordinary nutritional compensation will be required.

In our nation's history, it may have been possible at one time to accomplish our objective by diet alone, but that day is long past, due to the agricultural practices that have become the norm. The fact of the matter is that the quantity of the nutrients that we require are no longer available in the soil. They have effectively been "farmed" out of the soil and, as a result, are severely depleted in the fruits and vegetables that grow in it.

A landmark study done at the University of Texas at Austin by Donald Douglass and his team of researchers from the Department of Chemistry and Biochemistry was published in December 2004 in the *Journal of the American College of Nutrition*. They studied the US Department of Agriculture's nutritional data from both 1950 and 1999 for forty-three different vegetables and fruits. They found "reliable decline" in the amount of protein, calcium, phosphorus, iron, riboflavin, and vitamin C over the past half century, which the Douglass study attributed to the preponderance of agricultural practices designed to improve yield.

The Organic Consumers Association cites several other studies with similar findings. A Kushi Institute analysis of nutrient data from 1975 to 1997 found average calcium levels in twelve fresh vegetables dropped 27 percent; iron levels dropped 37 percent; vitamin A levels dropped 21 percent; and vitamin C levels dropped 30 percent. Another study revealed that one would have to consume eight oranges of those grown today to obtain the same amount of vitamin A that our grandparents got from one.

Still another aspect of nutrient availability in food is the often-ignored amount of nutritive loss as a result of freshness. On average, most produce loses 30 percent of nutrients within three days of harvest. What that may mean concerning the produce section of our grocery stores can only result in wonderment concerning how many nutrients are available to the consumer by the time the product finally becomes available for purchase.

A University of California study shows that vegetables can lose 15 to 55 percent of vitamin C in a week. Some spinach can lose 90 percent of nutritive value within the first twenty-four hours after harvest.

We will have a lengthy discussion on how to correct your deficiencies of a lifetime and to do so remarkably well. It is my intention at this time to reveal that attempting to make those corrections by eating a "healthy" diet alone will not be possible and is destined to result in failure.

STEP 2: REMOVE ALL TOXICITIES

In a very real sense, the accumulation of toxic substances in the human body in general and in the eye in particular is the antithesis to nutritional deficiencies. With respect to the normal function of human tissue, if you have too little of something you vitally require for the body to function optimally, you cannot be surprised when the body refuses to perform in the optimal manner and, as a result, the diseases of aging commence.

The opposite is also true. If you have too much of something, especially when that something is a toxic substance like a heavy metal or chemical, the intricate metabolic systems in the tissues cannot function. They are so mired down in the toxic sludge that the cells in a specific organ just shut down. You can supply a truckload of healthy nutrients, but the detrimental effect of those toxic substances prevents normal function to such an extent that it is like not having supplied the nutrients at all.

It has been my observation that patients are quick to realize the importance of an optimal diet, and the vast majority of them have realized early on that their doctors do not possess the skills to help. That awareness has been weathered well, however, because the vast majority of them have the competency to make those choices on their own. There are resources available either on the Internet or through local personnel to inform them, and health-food stores to support them in their mission to supply the body what is required to function optimally.

That enthusiasm and competency runs into a brick wall, however, when the patient decides their toxic burden is just as important as their diet in improving their overall general health, let alone in those groups of patients with a serious medical problem. The brick wall they encounter occurs when they come to understand that for them to become healthy, they will require their doctor to help. Only the doctor can order laboratory tests to identify those toxic substances and the prescription agents required to remove them once they are detected.

IT DEPENDS ON WHAT THE DEFINITION OF "IS" IS

Please excuse the President Clinton reference, but once again allow me to share a medical absurdity that will explain the brick wall I referred to earlier. Countless numbers of patients have approached their doctors after they have decided a toxic substance, usually a heavy metal, is responsible for why they feel so lousy. Mercury toxicity from dental amalgams is frequently the heavy metal referenced by the patient, but it could be any one of many metals, like cadmium, lead, or aluminum.

The doctor listens intently because the patient goes about explaining that they have had multiple mercury amalgam fillings in their mouth for many years. Amalgams, by definition, have a mercury content of at least 51 percent and are also described in the literature as leaching from the filling into the mouth and saliva. From there, the mere act of swallowing allows the mercury to be redistributed throughout the rest of the body. The doctor has been taught about heavy-metal toxicity during his medical education, so he still is comfortable enough with the conversation to let it continue.

The patient pleads with their doctor to order some lab tests that will allow the patient to confirm that mercury toxicity is responsible for their medical dilemma. Usually after multiple requests, it is possible for the doctor to finally agree to order the blood test by prescription to identify the presence of the offensive toxic substance. The patient feels good about having convinced the doctor to order the test. The doctor is willing to explore that mercury may be responsible for the patient's complaint. When the results of the test are finally available, the diagnosis becomes unavoidable. The lab results state that there is no mercury detectable in the blood specimen at all.

This scenario plays itself out multiple times per day throughout the United States. Allow me to point out the tragic error that has just been committed. What the patient could not have known is that in a doctor's training, the only form of metal toxicity the profession recognizes is acute toxicity.

In a case of acute toxicity, the offensive agent responsible for the patient's symptoms will always be found in the blood. A child who eats paint chips from lead-based paint, for instance, is loaded with lead. That lead is easily identified in the blood. Mercury toxicity due to amalgam fillings is not an acute toxic phenomenon. In those cases, the moment mercury enters the body, the cells of the body immediately take up the substance within the very matrix of the tissue, and there it will stay until extraordinary measures are employed to remove it.

At this point, it is safe to say that the only place in the entire body that will not demonstrate any smidgen of mercury is in the blood. The mercury is "locked-up" in the tissue. To identify a chronic exposure of any heavy metal, you must first administer a substance that pulls the offensive metal from the tissue into the blood and then assay the patient's urine because the kidney will remove that metal from the blood as it passes through the organ.

Chronic heavy-metal toxicity is devastating, and it plays an important role in causing eye diseases. These metals must be identified and removed to allow the eye to function normally once again.

This little-known and little-understood concept of chronic versus acute toxicity creates a large divide that cannot be traversed by the conventional medical doctor. As a patient, you can talk until you are blue in the face about how heavy metals can create a devastating effect on the normal functioning in the human body and still not be found in the blood, but it just will not matter. Your doctor cannot and will not be able to reconcile why a blood test cannot confirm heavy-metal toxicity.

You will require the assistance of a medical doctor who understands the definition of chronic heavy-metal toxicity and not only how to measure it but also how to correct it. With the kind of testing that is available, this can easily be done at home. The urine specimen can be sent to one of many special laboratories to monitor your progress as you continue to remove the metal and its influence on your eye disorder.

Step 1 and Step 2 have now been presented conceptually. The specifics of how to produce the changes required will be discussed in up-and-coming chapters in both cases. We now turn to Step 3, which I believe should be equally as interesting as the two that have preceded it and allow us to complete the treatment trilogy.

STEP 3: OPTIMIZE PERFUSION

It is more than likely that you have understood the limitations in conventional treatment of your eye disorder. That treatment, with little exception, is to do nothing at all. If you are just arriving at that level of awareness, the alternative world extends an open hand to welcome your arrival. There are many of you who recognized the limitations a long time ago and have developed treatment relationships with alternative practitioners in your area of the country.

The first two steps of the Three-Step Program are universally appreciated by all clinicians represented in the integrative domain. It is not an accident that you immediately felt comfortable with your alternative doctor, no matter if he was a chiropractor, naturopath, homeopath, osteopath, or medical doctor because he just talked differently than your eye doctor. The theme of your discussions should have closely resembled what we are discussing at this juncture in our conversation, which is the need to correct deficiencies and toxicities that have accumulated over a lifetime.

As good as these practitioners are at understanding and manipulating the human body to correct the two common elements we have just described, they unfortunately ignore the third. I am not sure if they actually ignore the third step because in my discussions with many of my colleagues, it appears they listen with great interest. They ask many questions of me during the discussion. They share their acknowledgment that the strategies I have developed add a dimension to restoring health. When that discussion has concluded, they leave me with the impression that they too will consider incorporating these modalities in their own practices.

The relationships with my medical colleagues have remained cordial and ongoing, but I must tell you that to date, I am not aware of any of my doctor friends who have taken our discussion to the next step in their own practices. I will continue to encourage them to do so in the future and hope that our future dialogue remains as beneficial as it has in the past.

While the discussions with my colleagues have remained theoretical, the rewards of optimizing perfusion are experienced on a daily basis by the individuals who follow my instruction to optimize their perfusion. These patients appear to appreciate a simple fact. If you wish to have an organ or any tissue in the human body work at its highest level of efficiency, you must provide a maximum amount of blood flow to that tissue. The blood is the medium by which nutrients are delivered and toxic waste products are disposed of.

It is just a fact that as we age, the vascularity of any region of the body decreases. With that decrease in blood flow, the pathologies of aging can ensue. Your own eye disorder has occurred as a direct result of this loss of blood flow and cannot be reversed unless it is restored.

The circulatory system consists of the heart and blood vessels.

There are two main divisions of blood vessels:

1. The arterial system. Arteries are the blood vessels that carry blood away from the heart and bring a blood supply to the tissues.

2. The venous system. These are the blood vessels that carry waste products, including toxic waste, away from the tissues and back to the heart for delivery to the organs of elimination.

The modalities that optimize perfusion that will be described greatly optimize perfusion in both kinds of blood vessels. You really cannot improve blood flow in only one type of blood vessel without having a similar improvement in the other.

In my explanation, I routinely emphasize arterial blood flow. Just keep in mind that they are equally important. Without an adequate blood flow, no nutrients can reach your cells, and no toxic substances can be removed. It should suffice to say you can take a truckload of nutrients and supplements, but if they cannot be delivered to the diseased tissue in your eye, it is as though you did not take them at all. That omission now stands to be corrected. Blood flow will be reestablished. Diseased tissue will be revived and nurtured back to healthy function once again.

IT'S THE MICROVASCULATURE, STUPID

I have already cited references to our past president on a number of occasions, and I cannot avoid the temptation to do it one final time. When he ran for the presidency in 1992, a member of his staff hung a sign in his Little Rock, Arkansas, headquarters that read, "It's the economy, stupid." The sign was intended to alert the campaign staff of the message they should not lose sight of when trying to convince voters to elect their nominee.

They transmitted the message to the public so well that the phrase has been etched in the memory of many who lived through that election to this very day. I intend no disrespect to the reader by employing a similar way to convey a message to those who are intent on restoring their lost vision. I have pulled it from my own memory and have now changed it slightly. It is my hope that it wears well with you and will call to mind the component of the Three-Step Program that ensures the success you are seeking to correct your eye disorder.

To appreciate the enormity of the microvasculature, let me ask a rhetorical question. If I could secure an artery from your big toe with a hemostat (similar to a pair of pliers), and then start to walk away in such a fashion so as to unravel you of all of your arteries (I am not talking about your veins—for our purposes, we will leave that system intact for the moment), how far would I walk before I have unwound all of them from the body?

The answer to the question is that I would have to walk over 140,000 miles, which is equivalent to multiple times around the equator to complete the task. Just think about that for a moment. How can that be so? Please allow me to explain.

Large arteries—and there are plenty of them—branch off the aorta (the main artery in the body) and start dividing. One artery branches into two. The two branch into four. The four branch into eight, sixteen, thirty-two, and so on. After an exponential branching has occurred, the artery makes its final branch and becomes a network of tiny, microscopic arteries that are not even visible with the naked eye. The structure at that point of the artery is called an arterial capillary. It is the most important blood vessel in the human body. If arterial capillaries could be placed from end to end, they would traverse the 140,000-mile distance that has been documented by science. It is truly miraculous to even be able to comprehend such enormity.

It is the accumulation of these microscopic arteries that collectively comprise the microvasculature. It is that microvasculature that brings a blood supply to nourish every nook and/or cranny of the human body. The reason they are so important is that they are the only blood vessels that come into an intimate proximity of a cell. The arterial capillaries have openings within their thin membranes, which allow oxygen, nutrients, vitamins, and minerals to exit the blood to enter into a single cell where those nutrients can be used to maintain or revive cellular function.

You do not lose any of your large arteries as you age, even though they restrict blood flow due to deposits of plaque that organize within them. On the other hand, you lose miles and miles of your microvasculature with advancing age. Once these tiny blood vessels are lost, they will not return on their own. It will require a combination of modalities to rescue them. We will describe those modalities in great detail in the up-and-coming chapters.

The Three-Step Program has now been presented in its most generalized format. My intention is to give you an opportunity to appreciate that you can do this. More than likely, you have already started. If so, I commend you for your initiative.

I will assist you in any way you feel you need encouragement and guidance. If you are at the beginning of this mission, nothing really changes. You need only to decide to initiate your program now, and you will be able to obtain similar results in record time by following the Three-Step Program.

As you read through the next chapters, the specifics of the program will be explained. Find the starting point that is the most comfortable for you. You can begin the moment you make the decision to do so. If you wish to become a part of the Three-Day Program, we may have the opportunity to meet face to face.

Whether you employ the components of this program in your home or in our office, the benefits to you will be substantial while following the Three-Step Program to regain your sight.

CHAPTER 6

THE THREE-STEP PROGRAM TO REGAIN YOUR SIGHT

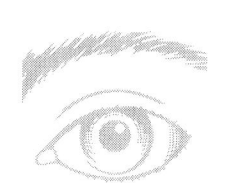

STEP 1: CORRECTING NUTRITIONAL DEFICIENCIES

The case has been made in prior chapters that the diseases of the eye, and most particularly those associated with advancing age, are due to the accumulated lack of nutrients over a lifetime. For the tissues of the eye to function again, those deficiencies must be corrected.

I have also been adamant about the fact that at this time of our agricultural evolution, you will not be able to correct these deficiencies through diet alone. Foods are so nutritionally poor that you cannot even be expected to maintain optimal health if you hypothetically started by being completely healthy to begin with.

In the case of those individuals with eye diseases that are manifestations of nutritional deficiencies, that theoretical state of health has been long left behind. The only individuals that continue to cling to the belief that you can restore health through diet alone appear to be members of the profession known as dietitians.

Local, state, and federal agencies codify by regulations that dietitians must be on the staff of all hospitals, schools, and nursing homes. They are the only healthcare professionals licensed to assess, diagnose, and treat nutritional problems. As for how effective they are at what they do, I should only need to mention that the dinner tray brought to you as a patient in any hospital in the country was created by the registered dietitian (RD) of that institution.

The final point about an RD that should allow me to put the topic of eating your way to health to rest is the fact that dietitians as a profession do not believe supplementation with vitamins, minerals, and other nutrients is necessary at all. The dietitian approach is directly opposite to my own.

For that reason, I will not take this opportunity to debate it. It should suffice to say again that if you have been hospitalized at some time in your life or can remember the meals that were made available to you in your cafeteria line at lunchtime, they were all brought to you through the courtesy of a dietitian. Without any further words that need to be spoken, I rest my case.

THE ROLES OF AN OPTIMAL DIET

Your personal dietary choices have evolved over a lifetime. Your likes and dislikes are unique to you. They result from the impact of many factors, not the least of which were culturally, ethnically, and economically determined. It just does not make sense to think that even with your vision on the line, someone should dictate to you what your diet should consist of when this so-called "evolutionary diet" is as much a part of you as your height, eye color, or hair color.

All too frequently, your best intention is to embrace the good suggestions and fashion a new dietary regime, and it usually only results in a return to your own evolutionary diet that is comprised of those components that you are the most comfortable with. Ultimately, all of these well-intended dietary recommendations result in not changing your diet at all.

Rather than insisting that your diet needs to change, it is my opinion that by obeying a few simple rules, you can eat "healthy" again and do so within the context of your evolutionary diet. The reason these dietary rules are so potent is that when they are followed, your food choices no longer will carry any potential to harm you. By eliminating the detrimental aspects of your personal choices, your evolutionary diet becomes the healthy one you have been searching for.

It all comes down to making intelligent choices in the quality of food you buy, not the actual foods themselves. These rules have as their ultimate objective an ability to make your evolutionary diet health promoting instead of health eroding.

Rule 1: Eat Organic

The majority of those who are suffering from the eye diseases of advancing age are members of the baby boomer generation. In yet another odd twist of fate, the vast majority of foods we were raised on met the checklist of organic foods already.

The definition of organic food is food that is grown without the use of pesticides, synthetic fertilizers, sewage sludge, genetically modified organisms, or ionizing radiation. For animal products such as meat, poultry, eggs, and dairy products to qualify as organic, these animals must not have been given antibiotics or growth hormones.

If you think about it, in large measure that definition describes our agriculture and livestock industries that were in their own evolutionary process in the 1940s and early 1950s. At some point, organic lost and the need to increase yield became the operational battle cry of the food-producing industry. From that point forward, foods may have looked the same but were certainly a vector to allow very toxic substances to gain an entry point into the body with the potential for devastating repercussions.

The food industry, along with federal agencies, continues to try to convince the public that there is no difference between conventionally grown fruits and vegetables and their organic counterparts. They are, however, losing the argument, and organic farming is having a resurgence of willing farmers to meet the demands of the consumers that make their opinions known by their pocketbooks.

Even though organic foods cost more, their popularity continues to demonstrate a new trend to return to naturally grown. The food industry is not taking this new demand well. They continue to obstruct any new regulation that easily allows the consumer to distinguish between the two forms of food available in the marketplace. They instead rely on the consumer to opt for the cheaper prices of conventionally grown food to dictate the decision on what type of food will be purchased.

Do not look for transparency in labeling any time soon to help in this matter, but there is a way to cut through the mystery by what is known as a PLU coding system.

The PLU codes are not a part of the food industry or the US Department of Agriculture. They are four- or five-digit numbers that appear as a small sticker adhered to each individual fruit or vegetable. The supermarkets have used them since 1990 to make checkout and inventory control easier, faster, and more accurate. They ensure that consumers pay the correct price by removing the need for cashiers to identify the product as being either conventionally or organically grown.

You as the consumer can easily identify the type of produce by visually checking the number which appears on each individual item. In short, a five-digit code that begins with the number eight signifies a genetically modified product. A five-digit code beginning with nine identifies an organically grown product. A four- or five-digit code beginning with a zero marks a nonqualified conventionally grown product.

You now have two ways to identify organic foods. If the food carries the USDA seal of "certified organic," the producer has applied to the USDA for permission to use the label after having met the rigorous standards set by that agency for that designation. The second way for you to identify the type of produce you are considering is through the use of the four- or five-digit PLU codes used by the supermarket industry to keep track of inventory and pricing at the checkout counter.

Between the two methods, you should find shopping a unique experience to assist you in your quest to pursue a healthy diet and still allow you to maintain the presentation and preparation you enjoy.

Rule 2: Avoid GMOs

In 1993, Monsanto set out to accomplish that which had never been done before: alter the DNA of a vegetable in such a way so as to allow the yield of a product to surpass industry expectations that had not been possible previously.

Monsanto elected corn as the first product to be altered in such a way. The objective was to change the DNA of the corn so it could withstand greater amounts of highly toxic pesticide. What resulted was a type of corn that when it was sprayed with pesticide would kill the larva of worms that resided under the cornhusk and that were previously rejected by the consumer when they selected the ears of corn at purchase. It is the reason that the paper bag still remains at the corn selection table of your supermarket today. Try as you might, you will not find any worms upon inspection.

Altering the DNA of a natural substance by its very suggestion is difficult to defend, but Monsanto and the farmers that used the seeds provided to them through the new "franken" corn continue to insist there is no need for concern.

If their argument in favor of genetic modification resonates with you, then so be it. In my opinion, following the golden rule of "Don't mess with Mother Nature" is worthwhile. Creating a product that can withstand higher levels of toxic pesticide is not a good thing to have as a final objective.

Newer forms of corn that have been genetically modified have been altered to include an insect-killing gene. GMO corn is a product that, no matter how good it may look, should have a skull and crossbones etched on every husk. The steadfast rule for you to follow is to avoid all GMO foods in your diet.

The bigger problem is that there are many more foods Monsanto has altered genetically, so you have to be careful not to become so complacent as to think of corn alone.

Here is a correct list of all genetically modified foods that exist in the marketplace today:

- corn
- soybeans
- sugar beets
- potatoes
- tomatoes
- squash
- golden rice
- salmon
- rapeseed
- honey
- cotton

- sugarcane
- flax
- papaya
- cottonseed oil
- peas
- dairy products
- vitamins

Rule 3: Do Not Avoid Meat

I have at least caught your attention by announcing that I certainly do not discourage eating meat. To be even more accurate, I actually encourage eating animals and animal by-products when the source of the animal in question has met some standards to allow it to qualify as healthy.

We have only to look at organized medicine and the "animal fat" craze initiated by it in the latter part of the 1900s to identify the origin of the avoidance of animal fat.

According to the explanation, the ingestion of animal fat was the root cause of cardiovascular disease for sure and probably of most of the other diseases as well. This manner of thinking led to the food industry supplying a number of low-fat and fat-free products that made it to our store shelves over a twenty-year span.

In another famous example of an odd twist of fate, these products, in order to compensate for a loss of taste, called upon the addition of the real cause of disease—carbohydrate—to fill the void. The fat-free products tasted much better. The consumer, feeling that they were complying with their doctor's wishes, got fatter. The food industry got richer, and disease underwent the greatest meteoric rise in such a brief period of time as has been recorded in the history of the modern world.

The livestock industry developed its own questionable practices. They fed their animals unusual quantities of grains (concentrated carbohydrates) to fatten them. They also laced that feed with antibiotics, supposedly to decrease infectious disease, and then initiated a program of injecting growth hormone so the animals would increase their muscle mass. All three of these measures produced livestock that yielded higher-valued, heavier animals at slaughter. Unfortunately, the consumer received a tainted and toxic product as a result.

It is not the meat or animal-fat consumption that is the problem. The problem is the toxic load that livestock acquires as a result of an industry that has little safeguards and oversight by governmental agencies, and there does not appear to be any time in the near future for that to change.

Just as you have been shown that you can have a healthy diet by eating organic fruits and vegetables, you can do the same when it comes to meat consumption—eat organic. Federal regulation for organic livestock certification requires the following:

- The animal must be raised on certified organic land.

- The animal must be fed organic feed free from antibiotics, growth hormones, animal by-products, pesticides, and chemical fertilizers.

- No antibiotics or growth hormone can be administered.

- The animal must have outdoor access.

I can now return to my opening to this section, which was the announcement that you do not and should not have to avoid meat. Let me go one step further by suggesting that organically raised, free-range, grass-fed livestock, particularly beef livestock, can actually qualify as a health food.

We will start that explanation by first discussing human anatomy. A human being has one stomach, and the digestive process essentially begins within it.

The fruits and vegetables in our diet contain varying amounts of fiber, which is quite difficult or almost impossible to digest. Because of that difficulty, they leave the stomach virtually unaltered.

Much of the vitamin and mineral content of these fruits and vegetables reside within the fiber component of the product and pass through the entire digestive system virtually untouched whereupon they are presented to the colon for elimination.

It is a fact that we select vegetables based on their fiber content to assist in promoting elimination, especially in those who may suffer from constipation. It cannot be ignored, however, that because of the fact that vitamins and minerals contained in fruits and vegetables leave the body untouched, the nutritional benefit from them is, at best, minimal due to their fiber content.

In the animal world, beef livestock anatomically possess four stomachs, which contribute to an extremely long digestive transit time. Along that journey, full digestion of all fiber-containing vegetable products is complete. As a result, the full nutrient content of whatever was consumed by the animal is made available throughout the entire carcass of the animal.

It is because of this anatomical and physiological fact that eating beef, and in particular organic beef, is one of the few ways to obtain an abundance of naturally derived, fully assimilable vitamins and minerals through eating meat. It is for this reason that I often refer to a cow or steer as a walking salad bar.

Rule 4: Shop the Periphery

It is no accident that virtually every supermarket has the same layout. The perishables are always along the outside walls, and the nonperishables are found in the various aisles on the inside of the store. Freshness and expiration dates really matter to the grocery store, and a constant vigilance to those items ensures patrons that their safety is kept as a number-one concern.

Concerning the food that makes it to the inside of the store, a different ball game is in play. In these processed foods, shelf life means everything. The chemicals employed to extend that shelf life are to be avoided at all costs. You can and should become a label reader. Except for an occasional item in the frozen section, you will need a degree in chemistry to read those labels.

Here is a list of the ten most common food additives to avoid:

1. Artificial sweeteners. Whether the packet is blue, pink, or yellow, you are exposing yourself to aspartame (NutraSweet), sodium saccharine (Sweet'N Low), or sucralose (Splenda). Rather than describing the ways these sugar substitutes can adversely affect you, it seems that a much better use of this effort is to give you an idea of what sugar substitutes you should consider that do not have the potential side effects of the previously mentioned three items.

   - Agave nectar

     0 calories

     The nectar is a product of the agave cactus with a taste and texture similar to honey. Agave is sweeter than sugar, so proponents suggest that you can use less to achieve a similar sweetness. It contains more fructose than table sugar, which according to a recent study is more likely to reduce your metabolism and insulin sensitivity.

   - Stevia leaf extract (Truvia)

     20 calories

     Derived from the Stevia plant and deemed to be the natural alternative to artificial sweeteners, refined Stevia products (Truvia) won approval by the FDA in 2008. It is sold in most grocery stores.

   - Sutalin

     12 calories

This was recently introduced by a company called Boresha and is a natural sweetener derived from white grape juice powder, pear fruit juice powder, and monk fruit extract.

2. High-fructose corn syrup (HFCS). HFCS is a highly refined artificial sweetener, which has become the number-one source of calories in America. It is found in almost all processed foods. HFCS puts the pounds on faster than any other ingredient. It increases your LDL (bad cholesterol) and contributes to the development of diabetes and tissue damage.

3. Monosodium glutamate (MSG). MSG is an amino acid used as a flavor enhancer in soups, salad dressings, chips, frozen entrees, and many restaurant foods. It is an excitotoxin, which is a substance that overexcites cells to the point of damage or death. It has been associated with depression, eye damage, fatigue, headache, and obesity.

4. Trans fat. Trans fats are used to enhance and extend shelf life of food products and are among the most dangerous substances you can consume. It is found in deep-fried fat foods and certain processed foods made with margarine or partially hydrogenated vegetables oils. Trans fats are known to increase the risk of heart attacks and strokes and to increase inflammation.

5. Common food dyes. Artificial coloring found in soda, fruit juices, and salad dressings are known to cause behavioral problems in children and lead to significant reduction in IQ. In animals, it has been linked to the development of cancer. The most offensive dyes are

- blue dye #1 and blue dye #2;

- red dye #3 (banned in 1950 for use in foods and cosmetics but continued to be used until supplies ran out); and

- yellow dye #6.

6. Sodium sulfite. This is a preservative used in winemaking and processed foods. According to the FDA, one in a hundred people is sensitive to sulfites in food. It is associated with asthma as well as headaches, breathing, and rashes. They have, in severe cases, led to death by provoking the anaphylaxis of the respiratory system.

7. Sodium nitrate / sodium nitrite. This is used as a preservative, coloring, and flavoring enhancer in bacon, ham, hot dogs, lunch meats, corned beef, smoked fish, and other processed meats. The ingredient, which sounds harmless, is highly carcinogenic once it enters the human digestive system. An attempt to ban it occurred by the USDA in 1970 but was vetoed by the food industry that claimed they had no alternative for preserving packaged meat products.

8. BHA and BHT. Butylated hydroxyanisole (BHA) and butylated hydroxytoluene (BHT) are preservatives found in cereals, chewing gum, potato chips, and vegetables oils. This preservative keeps food from changing color or flavor or becoming rancid. The substances affect the neurological system of the brain, alter behaviors, and have the potential to cause cancer.

9. Sulfur dioxide. Sulfur additives are toxic, and in the United States, the FDA has prohibited their use on raw fruit and vegetables. Adverse reactions include bronchial problems, particularly in those who are prone to asthma, hypotension, flushing, tingling sensations, and anaphylactic shock. They are found in beer, soft drinks, dried fruit juice, wine, vinegar, and potato products.

10. Potassium bromate. This is an additive used to increase volume in some white flour, bread, and rolls. It is known to cause cancer in animals.

Shopping in the periphery of your supermarket will keep you clear of most but not all of these hazardous products. You must rely on the label reading to be your safety-check valve.

It goes without saying that buying and eating organic remains the goal. Just about all major grocery stores have a wide selection of products to choose from. You may even do better by visiting a local farmer and discussing their farming practices with them. They are fully aware of the organic food controversy and will be delighted to share their own knowledge of where organic farming is practiced in the area. While you are at it, ask about the available sources of organic livestock and visit them also. It will be time well spent.

Rule 5: Carbohydrates with Caution

Your diet, however varied it may be, only has three possible foods associated with it. Those three categories are the following:

1. Carbohydrates

2. Proteins

3. Fats

We have already addressed the subject of proteins in great depth in this section of the chapter devoted to encouraging you to eat organic meat products to actually obtain a greater amount of vitamins and minerals than you may have thought previously possible.

The discussion now turns to the role carbohydrates should play as a component of your healthy diet. To help you in that endeavor, it will serve us well to divide carbohydrates into two distinct groups:

1. Nutrient-sparse carbohydrates

2. Nutrient-dense carbohydrates

Over the last fifty years, a major shift in our diet has occurred that could not be compensated for in such a short span of time. It was the double whammy of the dawning of the fast-food industry and the exponential elevation of our carbohydrate consumption that has created the epidemic of type 2 diabetes. The baby boomer generation was the first to feel its effects. It continues to increase in the millennial generation to such a degree that, for the first time in human history, the generation that follows is expected to die sooner than the generation that preceded it.

The first hint that something new was brewing happened during the Vietnam and Korean War era when young men, eighteen to twenty years of age, were brought home in body bags to Dover, Delaware. When soldiers' remains are returned, many undergo a full autopsy no matter what the obvious cause of death was. It was during the autopsies on those soldiers that the first evidence of what was to come was detected.

Two studies that are frequently cited (70 percent in one and 48 percent in another) revealed the presence of advanced cardiovascular disease to such an extent not ever seen before even in an elderly population, let alone in a group of late adolescents. The arterial lesions and atherosclerotic plaque accumulation was the hallmark evidence of the damage to the vasculature in any diabetic. It just had never been seen before in a group of males that young.

The Vietnam veterans are now in their sixties and seventies. They now are the full-blown diabetics that the autopsies were able to forecast that many years in advance. They are the spearhead of the diabetic epidemic that is now in full display.

It is the constant barrage of elevated carbohydrate levels and the rapid and sustained blood-sugar levels that result that bring us to this point. A new disease has been born that is now out of control. It is carbohydrates in the diet that are to blame.

The form of diabetes we were most familiar with was a form known as type 1 diabetes. It usually begins in childhood and is the result of an autoimmune disorder. In type 1 diabetes, the pancreas cannot produce insulin in response to elevation in blood sugar. It is insulin that allows glucose to enter the cell. In type 2 diabetes, so much insulin is secreted that the tissues develop an insulin resistance. In both cases, blood sugars rise. The constant elevation of blood sugar referred to as glycemia damages all tissue it comes into contact with, and the heart and blood vessels become ground zero.

To protect you from sustained glycemia, the construction of your healthy diet should attempt to eliminate the nutritionally sparse carbohydrates while encouraging the nutritionally dense ones.

The nutritionally sparse carbohydrates are more accurately described as nutritionally absent. They contain little to no nutritional value. They break down during digestion and are converted into glucose in large quantities, which rapidly enter the bloodstream. This sudden elevation in blood sugar triggers the pancreas to produce and secrete large amounts of insulin that the cells eventually no longer respond to, leading to sustained blood-sugar elevations.

If you are a diabetic already, you must severely limit the carbohydrate content of your diet as part of your treatment. If you are not a diabetic yet, you can protect yourself from ever becoming a diabetic by doing the same.

The following foods are represented in the nutritionally absent group:

- sugar
- bread
- rice
- potatoes
- pasta
- fruit juices

- cereals

You can easily recognize a group of foods referred to as "the starches." The starches always pose a potential problem and should be eaten cautiously. They cannot be modified to reduce their blood-sugar elevation risk.

As an example, what I frequently hear from patients is something like, "I eat Ezekiel bread, not white bread," or "I eat wild rice or brown rice, not white rice." The fact of the matter is that a slice of Ezekiel bread, although it does have nutritional value, has the same number of carbohydrates as a slice of white bread. The color or other components do not matter. It is the carbohydrate content that matters. Even though some healthier versions of some of these representatives could be considered a healthier version, the carbohydrate content is what matters.

As emphatic as I have been with respect to consuming the starches—the nutritionally absent foods—I cannot encourage you enough to eat unlimited amounts of the nutritionally dense form of carbohydrates. Collectively, you know them as the vegetables. They are loaded with vitamins and minerals where the starches are not.

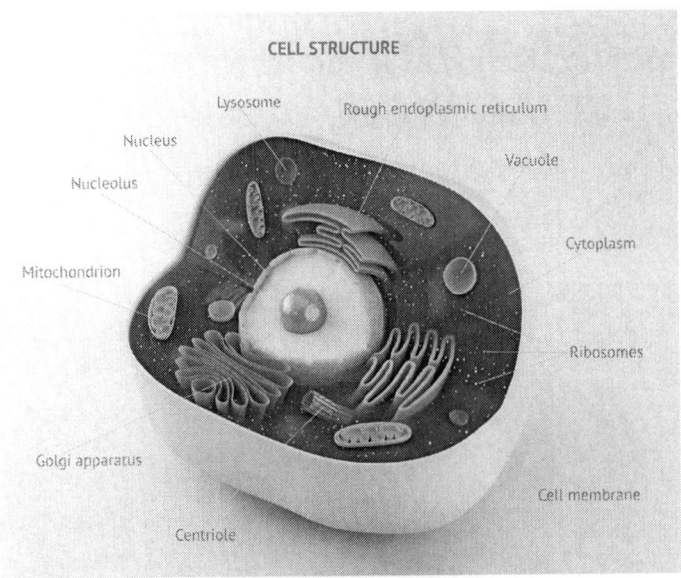

The biggest reason they can be recommended so enthusiastically is that the elevation in blood-sugar levels is, at best, only minimal. The pancreas is not overly stimulated. Consequently, insulin levels rise slowly. With that rise, the cells of the body can adjust to accommodate the influx of sugar into the cells.

Rule 6: Fats Are Your Friend

Fats, referred to scientifically as lipids, have been receiving a bad rap for years. Even though the volume has been lowered considerably by the conventional medical world, lipids just do not receive any respect. Allow me to do just that by explaining some newly discovered scientific facts that may allow you to pay a little respect to lipids.

You are made up of, on average, seventy trillion cells. Depending on each organ, cells have highly specific functions. A heart cell conducts electrical activity so as to be able to, in a synchronous manner, contract sixty to seventy times a minute every day for a lifetime. A kidney cell removes nitrogenous waste and excess water every second of your life for a lifetime. I could go on here, but you can see the idea.

Each of your seventy trillion cells is comprised of a cell membrane, which completely forms the boundaries of a cell, and a nucleus located in the center, which contains all of the genetic information required by the cell. The nucleus is suspended in a gel-like maze known as the cytoplasm. You can refer to a graphic interpretation of one cell, keeping in mind that you have about seventy trillion others.

Until only recently, all the respect has been directed at the nucleus as the most important part of a cell because it was understood that it controlled all the functions of each cell.

The first sign that the nucleus may not be all that important was as a result of an experiment where the nucleus of a cell was removed and, to the astonishment of the investigators, the cell lived on and carried on all of its functions without one single glitch. The only thing the cell could not do was divide and replicate. This was not that big of a surprise in that when the nucleus was removed, all the genetic material was also removed, and the DNA could not replicate. This same experiment was conducted many times and all met with the same result.

A different experiment was conducted by another group of scientists where the cell membrane was removed and the nucleus was left intact. The result of this experiment was that the entire cell died instantaneously. It does not take a PhD in biochemistry to figure out that the nucleus cannot be that important, and a cell membrane must be really important.

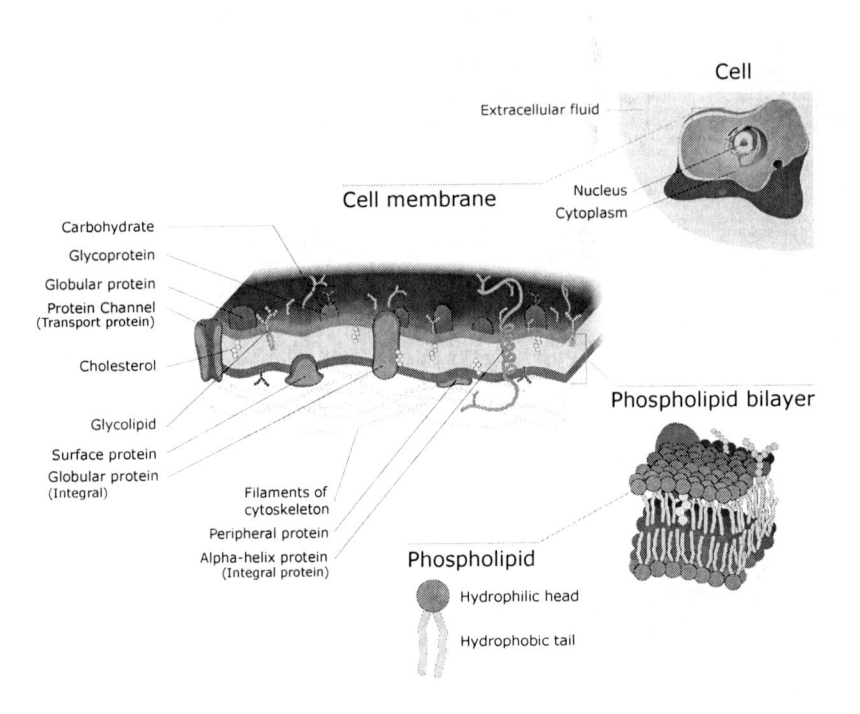

This startling discovery and the implications of it have been described by many, but a good description of this concept has been explained in a now-famous book written by Bruce Lipton, PhD, and is entitled *The Biology of Belief*. I recommend it if you would like to know more. The summation of the book on this issue is as follows.

The nucleus of a cell is the repository of information. It is the equivalent of a library or, in modern-day cyber language, the hard drive of a computer. As a hard drive, it may store information, but it is the cell membrane that acts as the keyboard. It supplies the directions and commands for all cell function. We need to talk about caring for the cell membrane in a way that ensures that those commands remain accurate, or it can result in cells that cannot function effectively because the membrane cannot function optimally.

Let's go back to those seventy trillion cells with the newest revelation that there are seventy trillion cell membranes that act as the keyboard to direct all the function within a cell. Each cell membrane is constructed as a bilipid membrane with one row of fatty acid comprising the outer membrane and another row of fatty acid comprising the inner membrane.

A fatty acid has a head at one end and two legs at the other. The outer layer of fat is oriented so that all the heads are facing to the outside of the cell. The inner layer of fatty acids is oriented with the heads pointing toward the inside of the cell.

All the legs of both the outer and inner leaflets of the cell membrane extend toward each other and closely approximate directly contacting one another. The composition of those leaflets is comprised of specific fats in equally specific quantities. Only when that specificity is achieved will the message sending of the cell membrane work flawlessly.

There are two main groups of fatty acids. One group is classified as omega-6, and the other group is known as omega-3. They are collectively referred to as "essential fatty acids" because they are not made by the body and must be supplied through the diet.

If the diet lacks any specific essential fatty acid of either the omega-6 or omega-3 group, the cell membrane cannot function optimally. In a very real sense, your keyboard sends confusing and unintelligent commands to the cell. It is your diet and the quality and quantity of the individual essential fatty acids that will determine the construction of your keyboard. It will be up to your daily fat consumption in the foods you select that will allow or inhibit the cell membrane to provide the messaging that will permit the cell to work as it was intended. If you do not, cell functions are disturbed, and the foundation for disease is laid.

Your seventy trillion cells are hardly immortal. They die off with varying speed. Some cells die off rapidly and are replaced by new cells rapidly. The cornea of the eye, for example, turns over every twelve hours. The cells of the lining of the gut have a life cycle of approximately thirty-six hours. Large nerves in the body have a life cycle of approximately ninety days. It is accurate to say that, at a minimum, you turn over at least seventy trillion cells every ninety days. The person reading this book in their comfy lounge chair did not even exist four months ago.

It is to be marveled that such a seamless replacement process occurs. How precise the replacement process will be is an enormous responsibility on your part with the diet you construct for yourself. The replication of your cells is a function of the nucleus and will occur without much ill effect produced by your diet selection. You only need to provide adequate calories to supply the energy for the cell to divide.

Once the DNA replication process begins, it is computer programmed to complete that process without any external forces that will alter it. The real potential for a problem is the fact that you turn over seventy trillion cell membranes every ninety days also. You will have to provide the raw material in the form of the essential fatty acids that are consumed through your dietary choices to make sure the construction of your seventy trillion keyboards are able to deliver commands to the cell function without error.

Of the three foods that you consume in your diet, the fat content in that diet is by far the most important. The "fat scare" era of the previous century and the remnants of it that remain to this very day are counterproductive. Eliminating fat from the diet to obtain a health benefit will result in cell dysfunction and disease. If you suffer from a disease, as long as that disease is not genetic, you can only recover from that disease by correcting the composition of your keyboard, otherwise known as your cell membrane.

Rule 7: Optimal Hydration for Health

The medium by which nutrients are transported throughout the body is a liquid one. The fluidity of the blood is conferred to it as a result of the water content of it. Varying degrees of dehydration limit the delivery of blood to the cell via small microscopic arterial blood vessels called capillaries. The capillary network was discussed earlier and will be addressed yet again in the following chapters of this book.

The blood is a delivery medium by which all nutrients arrive into the vicinity of a cell. It is like a package that is being sent to you that arrives at the vicinity of your ability to open it called your mailbox. You will have to take the necessary steps to take it into your home in order to open the package and utilize the contents found inside.

Analogous to your body's mailbox is the arterial capillary that delivers your nutritional package to its ultimate destination, which is a cell. To carry that package in the remaining short steps so that the contents can actually be utilized is a pure liquid medium known as the tissue fluid.

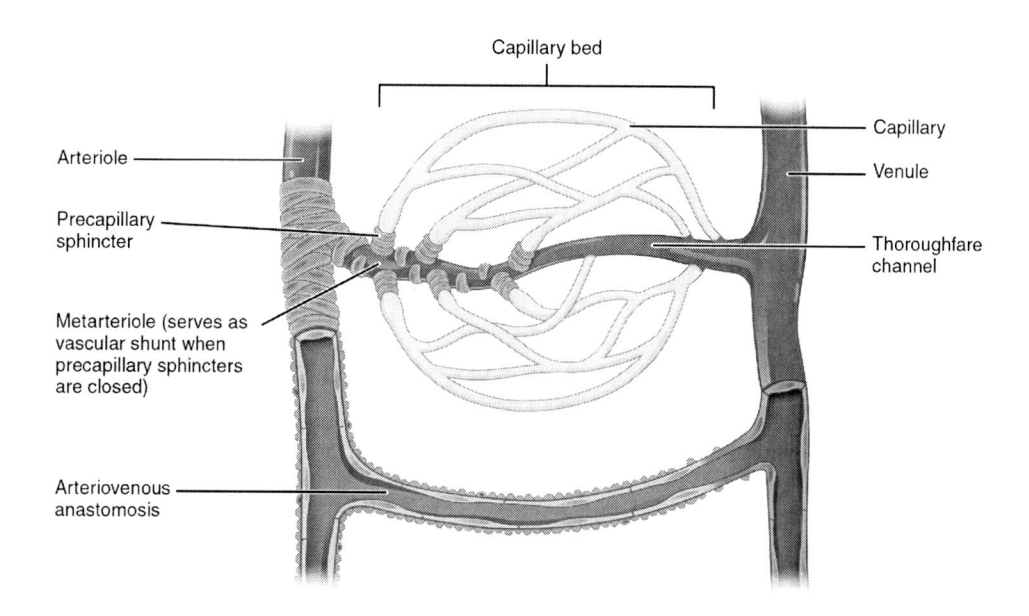

Tissue fluid is a clear, water-based fluid that makes the final delivery to the cell possible. After the cell has utilized the contents that have been delivered, various amounts of waste products need to be carried away from the cell to the curb where they can be carted off by a microscopic venous structure known as a venous capillary. Once again, the medium by which the refuse goes to the curb is the tissue fluid. Your hydration level allows that final transportation of either delivery or removal to be an easy process or a difficult one.

Yet a final function of optimal hydration is the contribution that your body's water content provides to a requirement to conduct electricity. All living beings are creatures that allow for the free flow of electrical energy. The ignition of that energy begins with the uniting of a sperm with an egg at conception and will not be extinguished until the hour of our death.

The movement of electrical energy throughout the body relies completely upon the individual's water content and a mixture of charged elements that can conduct electricity that collectively is referred to as an electrolyte solution. Tissue fluid on the outside of the cell and cytoplasm on the inside of the cell is the electrolyte solution of life.

Even though these complex physiological processes have been simplified for our purposes, they are an accurate explanation of the role of proper hydration in the human body. It is the tissue fluid and the water content of that fluid that allow the following to occur:

1. The delivery of nutrients to the cell

2. The removal of waste products away from the cell

3. The dynamic flow of electrical energy to circulate throughout the body

There are guidelines that, if followed, can allow you to meet the daily water requirements to achieve optimal hydration.

- You should drink one half of your body weight in ounces of water per day. That means if you weigh 150 pounds, you should drink at least 75 ounces of water a day.

- The word "water" means just that. It does not mean soda, tea, coffee, or any other drink that you may think of. The moment something is added to water, a chemical reaction occurs between the added substance and the water, forming a completely different compound.

- Tap water with all of its contaminants, both organic and inorganic, should be avoided as a water source. Public drinking-water systems brag about how sewer water can be treated so as to return it to drinking water at the end of the process. That image alone should be enough to allow you to avoid it.

- Bottled water may not be the answer either. In some cases, it is merely a glorified tap water put in a poorly constructed plastic bottle. These bottles leach caustic chemicals known as phthalates, which can by themselves lead to medical difficulties. If those bottles are allowed to sit in the sun, the heat that is generated actually causes the bottles to decompose.

- Let's face it. You need to filter your own water. At a minimum, there are sink-top units that do an acceptable job of purifying the water supplied to your home. A more expensive variation known as reverse osmosis (RO) water is probably the most reliable way to process your own water because of its ability to filter out contaminates. RO systems do such a good job of removing contaminants that they can remove beneficial minerals too. To compensate for this, a pinch of sea salt or Himalayan salt will bring your filtered water to a high-grade electrolyte solution.

THE COMPONENTS OF OPTIMAL SUPPLEMENTATION

From the beginning of the discussion, Step 1: Correcting Your Deficiencies, I have been clear that you will not be able to "eat your way" to optimal health. Since the beginning of this chapter, we have been describing how you can best construct your diet to come as close to optimal as possible, and even more importantly, how not to allow your diet selection to adversely affect your health.

It will be correct supplementation that will take you the rest of the way. It is more than likely accurate that you can supplement your way to health if we can assume that your diet selection will take you part of the way there. The best way to leave the optimization issue is that between the two, you will be able to accomplish your objective.

I have been practicing integrative medicine for over twenty years. In that period of time, the most frequently asked question by the patients I have consulted with has been, "Hey, Doc, what should I take?" Of course, the requested response was an attempt by the patient to find out what supplements I would recommend that could allow him to correct his deficiency status. The question was earnest and simple, and it was assumed I would provide him with a list of products he was willing to purchase upon my recommendation.

For at least seventeen of those twenty years, I could not bring myself to recommend any product that could put this question to rest. No matter what I would have suggested, the patient was poised to purchase. I was not pleased enough with and did not think enough of any product or product line to put my reputation behind it.

I know it would have been easy to decide on a group of products that had high-quality constituents and that the patient would certainly have benefited from having taken them. As you will soon have explained, those supplements would not have been optimal.

Due to the fact that my answer to the simple question about what supplements to take turned out to be my opportunity to educate patients on how to construct a supplement program, it is only proper for me to do the same for you. After that explanation concluded, my final instruction was to advise the patient to find a quality company that produced reputable supplements and that also had their reputation and integrity to protect.

Instead of a five-minute simple response by naming products, my discussion of the components of an optimal supplement program took forty-five minutes to an hour to complete. The time involved did not matter.

What did matter was that the patient left my office educated on the subject of supplementation in a way he never anticipated but that made him an enlightened consumer. From that point forward, he was capable of making choices concerning all supplements that allowed him to become a much better patient than he was before meeting me.

This teaching session became known as "The Six Basic Components of Any Supplement Program." It is presented to you now with the same intention in mind.

THE SIX BASIC COMPONENTS OF ANY OPTIMAL SUPPLEMENTATION PROGRAM

The following list of six components is considered to be a starting point in the formation of any supplement program. In those individuals who are healthy, these six components will maintain that state of health. For those patients with health challenges, additional supplements will initially be required to compensate for a deficient nutrient or group of nutrients. At some point, they will be able to maintain their optimal nutritional status by adhering to the six components that will now be described.

1. A good multivitamin product

This is the supplement that has caused me to have difficulty in recommending supplements to my patients. The first hurdle is that, except for only a few instances, the constituents of the vast majority of the supplements are all synthetic.

If you have any question as to whether your multivitamin is synthetic or not, turn the label around to expose the list of vitamins contained. If you need a degree in chemistry to read the label, you have confirmed that the components are synthetic.

I realize that the molecule that was formulated in the lab of the supplement company is the exact same molecule as the naturally occurring form. In my own mind, it is just not the equivalent of its natural counterpart and, for that reason, was difficult for me to recommend it.

To allow me to overcome my bias, there are companies that produce multivitamin supplements that are whole-food derived. The component vitamins were "alive" for sure at one time and might even continue to be alive today.

My problem with whole-food multivitamins is that there is no standardization to quantify the amount of each vitamin or, for that matter, what the total list of vitamins contained in the product actually is. When you inspect the label on the back of whole-food vitamins, you find words like "peppers," "radishes," "asparagus," etc. With farming practices as they are, what does that actually say about the quality and quantity of the contents?

There you have it. I then told the patient to pick one and go with a company known for it's high quality and select a good multivitamin to headline their supplement program.

2. Optimal macromineral supplement

These are minerals your body needs in larger amounts. They are usually never included in a multivitamin to the magnitude that is required and therefore will need to be supplemented separately. The following are the seven macrominerals:

- calcium
- potassium
- phosphorus
- chloride
- magnesium
- sulfur
- sodium

3. Optimal micromineral supplement

Microminerals are often referred to as "trace minerals." There are over eighty trace minerals that can be utilized in metabolic reactions in the body. They, like the macrominerals, are not found in a multivitamin and require an additional supplement to achieve optimal levels.

4. Optimal fatty-acid supplementation

You have probably noted how important fatty acids are in allowing the body to operate optimally from my earlier discussion about the importance of fat in the diet.

The entire concept of the role of fats is, at best, misunderstood and for the most part, ignored. The importance of fatty-acid replacement is so critical that it cannot and will not be corrected by diet alone. It will require its own supplementation program, which is just as important as the first three components are.

It is at this point that my patients reveal that they are taking fish oil, which they have been led to believe is the correct way to supplement for fatty-acid optimization.

Fish oil consists of two omega-3 fatty acids in approximately a fifty-fifty mixture:

- EPA: eicosapentaenoic acid
- DHA: docosahexaenoic acid

These are very complex omega-3 fatty acids and are not tolerated well by the body. They have gained their popularity because of their ability to decrease inflammation and, as a result, have been able to lessen pain associated with degenerative joint diseases such as rheumatoid and osteoarthritis. I will take up this matter a little further on in this book.

The point that should be made at this time is that fish oil does not correct fatty-acid deficiency. There are two reasons for this.

1. EPA and DHA are omega-3 fatty acids. They have no omega-6 supplementation potential.

2. Taking EPA and DHA fish oil is actually hazardous to your health (I will explain this later).

To accomplish supplementation to optimize the fatty-acid content of the body, there must be a blend of omega-6 and omega-3 essential fatty acids. For the longest time, even though the scientific community was aware of the need for a blend of omega-6 and omega-3, they did not know what that blend should be.

The breakthrough finally came in 1993 through the work of an Israeli physician by the name of Shlomo Yehuda. His published work in that year revealed two important scientific facts that finally allowed us to solve the fatty-acid supplementation query.

CHAPTER 6: THE THREE-STEP PROGRAM TO REGAIN YOUR SIGHT

The first of his findings finally determined the proper ratio of fatty acids required to optimally maintain the integrity of the cell membrane. He established a ratio of four to one of omega-6 fatty acids to omega-3 fatty acids. This was the first time we were able to see that we needed far more omega-6 fatty acids in replacing the essential fatty acids in the body than we did of the omega-3 type.

This finding by itself was monumental enough, but his work went even further. In his second revelation, he spelled out succinctly what oils should be consumed to supply the correct proportions of essential fatty acids.

He described these oils as foundation oils from which the body could then build the remaining necessary fatty acids of that lineage. As with building a house, starting with the right foundation allows you to end up with a sturdy home. So too, the foundation oil allows you to complete the task of correctly constructing your fatty-acid network.

The foundation oil in the omega-6 lines comes from a category of omega-6 fatty acids referred to as linoleic acid, and the two representative oils from that group are primrose oil and safflower oil. The foundation oil of the omega-3 line comes from a group of oils called alpha-linolenic acid. The two representative oils of that group are flaxseed oil and chia oil.

With this information available, the healthcare industry for the first time could develop the supplementation recommendations necessary to create the field of medicine that had been so lacking to that point. This message, unfortunately, did not ever reach the public, who continue to take fish oil under the illusion that "it must be right because my doctor told me to do it."

With Dr. Yehuda's description of a fatty-acid blend, a new dilemma was created. It does not make any practical sense to think that someone will mix a batch of oils at home to meet the standards created by him. There are two supplement companies that have taken that information and produced the products that will allow you to optimize your fatty-acid deficiency by purchasing a fatty-acid replacement product formulated with the knowledge of Dr. Yehuda's research. These are the two companies:

- www.BodyBio.com

  four-to-one oil

- www.Yes-Supplements.com

  ultimate EFA

5. Enzymes for optimal digestion

Nature provides in an uncanny way to take care of its own. Foods in nature contain the enzyme necessary for proper digestion and optimal assimilation and absorption of their nutrients into the blood.

When these foods are cooked, any proteins as well as naturally occurring enzymes are denatured and destroyed. In order to allow those nutrients to be absorbed into the bloodstream, you only need to take digestive enzymes that will take over when your foods cannot.

There are three foods that require additional enzyme assistance. By reading the label, you should look for the following:

- amylase: used to digest carbohydrates

- protease: used to digest proteins

- lipase: used to digest fats

You can usually find all three in a single product. Enzymes should be taken at every meal.

6. Optimal antioxidant potential

The battleground of life is played out at the cell membrane. It is here that chemical reactions occur with reactive oxygen species frequently referred to as "free radicals," which react and interfere with the activities that are carried out at the membrane itself.

These "oxidation reactions" damage the membranes, which as resilient to injury as they are, can still be overcome by that injury, lose their integrity, and allow cell death to ensue. Extracellular oxidation must be curtailed to permit a cell to undergo its full life cycle rather than abruptly succumbing to these potent oxidation forces.

Words are powerful, and opposing words can be equally powerful. If you wish to interfere with the forces of oxidation, you can prevent those forces from damaging the cell membrane by utilizing the power of antioxidation to carry out that task.

For the longest time, my go-to antioxidant of choice was vitamin C. It was inexpensive and effective. It was only a few years ago that the go-to antioxidant of choice became a naturally occurring carotenoid found in an algae known as haematococcus pluvialis known as astaxanthin.

One fact, and one fact alone, allowed the change in my choice to be rather easy to make. Here is that fact. One twelve-milligram capsule of astaxanthin has the antioxidant equivalency of seventy-two thousand milligrams of vitamin C. That is an unbelievable amount of firepower to protect cell membrane integrity.

A second fact concerning astaxanthin is that it has a half-life of twenty-three hours. Essentially, that means when you take your daily twelve-milligram dose at eight in the morning today, half of it is still active tomorrow morning at eight when you are scheduled to take your next dose.

SENSIBLE SUPPLEMENTATION

As I begin this section on supplementation, I want to make certain to point out that in those individuals afflicted with eye diseases, an elevated magnitude of supplementation would be required at the beginning of their supplement program. Dr. Edward Kondrot created a number of high-potency proprietary formulas that he has developed to meet the deficiency states most associated with eye diseases. I fully endorse Dr. Kondrot's supplement program and encourage you to consider his products on my website, www.PittsburghEye-Protocol.com.

At some point, it is appropriate to assume that you have corrected your deficiencies and should be able to "dial back" the intensity of your supplementation program. At that point, you may want to consider pursuing what I refer to as "sensible supplementation" to maintain every bit of nutritional gain but simplify the daily program of supplements that you require. I will now describe the program I use in my practice and explain how that evolution occurred.

WHAT SHOULD I TAKE?

This conversation on supplementation began with the revelation that during the first seventeen years of my practice, I felt that I could not in good conscience recommend a product line for my patients to use when I personally could not use the products myself. Four years ago, that all changed with the introduction of a product called F3.

The game changer (as I came to know the product better) is that F3 is neither synthetic nor a whole-food extract. Instead, F3 is a combination of three algae grown in hydroponically controlled environments under organic cultivation protocols.

These algae have been selected for their nutritional content and other unique properties from over eight thousand species. Their selection was so appropriate and the science so compelling that my medical practice has been drastically changed when it comes to the supplement I recommend.

Even though the algae source alone was important to me, because it was neither synthetic nor whole food, the most relevant fact regarding F3 was that it was able to accomplish all of the six components of my extensive supplement program in one single supplement alone. That's right. F3 contains optimal quantities of all vitamins, macrominerals, trace minerals, essential fatty acids, enzymes, and antioxidants in one capsule. It is the only way that I know to receive the components of all six supplements rolled up into one fully organic product.

As arduous as the previous six-item program was to follow, the patients still did so. Their intention was to get better, and they followed my recommendations even though the program was costly. With the advent and emergence of F3, a new banner is displayed on our supplement program, which is now referred to as "sensible supplementation."

Sensible supplementation has three components:

1. F3: This is the workhorse and foundation of six supplements in one; it is easy to take, organic, and 100 percent fully assimilable.

2. Four-to-one oil: Even though all omega-6 and omega-3 oils are in F3, they are not present in a ratio of four-to-one as described by Yehuda. One tablespoon of the oil per day is all it takes to keep membrane health at optimum.

3. Astaxanthin: There is already astaxanthin in F3, but this twelve-milligram capsule that is taken daily boosts antioxidant protection so well that it is equivalent to taking seventy-two thousand milligrams of vitamin C.

There is a Three-Step Program to regain your sight. We have just provided the reference information for the first step of the Three-Step Program.

Do not allow the accumulation of so much information frighten you. This entire chapter can be reduced to just one simple phrase: "Step 1: Correct all deficiencies."

CHAPTER 7

REMOVING YOUR TOXICITIES

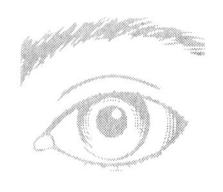

Having just described how the deficiencies of a lifetime finally impact the body's ability to function normally, it should come as no surprise that the opposite problem, having too much of anything, will have the potential to be equally harmful. This becomes even more obvious if the substance in excess has been scientifically established as toxic.

In our teenage and early adult years, this toxic burden is usually well tolerated, especially when it is slowly accumulated. A metabolic "workaround" by the body to compensate for the offensive substances permit biochemical pathways to proceed virtually unaffected. What is blatantly obvious, however, is that at some point, the workarounds are no longer possible, and a foothold for the initiation of disease ensues.

The diseases of advancing age collectively provide the culmination of a lifetime of accumulated toxins. There is not any system of the body that can escape the consequences of toxicity. Some regions are more vulnerable than others. If the substance is inhaled, a compromise of respiratory function can be anticipated. If the substance is leached from mercury amalgam fillings, the harmful effects are distributed to other body regions by either swallowing it or by having the mercury travel through a three-millimeter plate of bone through the roof of the mouth to gain access to the brain.

The important message is that these toxic substances can be identified and eliminated. It is possible to quantify the amount of the offensive agents that are actually retained within the body. Once quantified, we can easily follow the success of our detoxification program through repeat testing. There are pharmaceutical and nondrug compounds that can assist in removing the toxic load that has accumulated over a lifetime.

There is a plan that can be followed to remove the toxic burden from your body in order to take you to your intended goal. Removing the toxic burden will require you to follow that plan. Let's take a look at the components of such a plan and present the options that assure the greatest likelihood for success. You can restore your lost vision—*now*—and, by removing all of your toxicities, be able to regain your sight once again.

WHAT ARE THE TOXINS?

There are numerous classification methods to facilitate a discussion of the toxic burden of the body. In previous chapters on food and nutrients, many of these toxic substances have already been discussed. The care and precautions you incorporate into the selection of foods and water can eliminate any additional entry points for further contamination of body tissue. The general rule of "eating organic" and drinking purified and filtered water is your best insurance policy to prevent additional entrance into the body of these harmful substances.

Our next discussion will need to focus on how to rid the body of the toxic load that has already taken up residence within the tissues. The most problematic toxins that alter tissue function are referred to as the heavy metals. These toxic materials accumulate over a lifetime and profoundly and adversely affect tissue function by interfering with the metabolic processes of a cell and its cell membrane. There is not any body tissue or organ that is spared the wrath of these metals, and they are considered enemy number one on your to-do list to regain your sight.

The following is a list of the most recognized and commonly detected heavy metals:

antimony	cobalt	platinum
beryllium	copper	silver
boron	lead	thallium
cadmium	manganese	tungsten
chromium	mercury	zinc
	nickel	

The exposure to these heavy metals varies with an individual's geography, food and water source, occupation, and other environmental factors. Some of the most injurious exposure comes from medical and dental intervention, which, once again in an odd twist of fate, incriminates these two healthcare entities as the provocateur and not the eradicator of disease.

THE EFFECTS OF HEAVY METALS

There is no organ or body system that is resistant to the harmful effects of heavy-metal exposure. The root of entry more than likely is the major determining factor in what organ will be most affected with the contamination, but certain body tissues demonstrate a predilection toward being influenced by specific metals and resistant to others.

The following list is comprised of the most common heavy metals associated with human tissue dysfunction and disease. The list should be preceded by this salient point: eye diseases can result from chronic exposure to any of them. Also included are the most common sources of heavy-metal exposure associated with each.

arsenic: associated with bronchitis, dermatitis, poisoning

cadmium: kidney damage, lung disease, lung cancer, bone defects like osteomalacia and osteoporosis, GI disorders

lead: mental retardation in children, developmental delay, fatal infant encephalopathy, congenital paralysis, neural deafness, and acute or chronic damage to the nervous system (Dr. Ed Kondrot references that lead is the number-one heavy metal he has detected that leads to eye disease.)

manganese: causes damage to the nervous system (via inhalation or contact)

mercury: tremors, gingivitis, psychological changes, acrodynia caused by pink hands and feet, damage to the brain and nervous system

zinc: causes corrosive effect on the skin and damage to the nerve membrane (via fumes)

chromium: damage to the nervous system along with fatigue and irritability

copper: anemia, liver and kidney damage, along with stomach and intestinal damage

Sources of Exposure

arsenic: pesticides, fungicides, metal smelters

cadmium: welding, electroplating, pesticides, fertilizer, cadmium, nickel batters, nuclear fission plants

lead: paint, pesticides, smoking, automobile emissions, mining, burning of coal

manganese: welding, fuel additives

mercury: pesticides, batteries, paper industry, dental intervention

zinc: refineries, brass manufacturing, metal plating, plumbing

chromium: mines, mineral sources

copper: mining, pesticide production, chemical industry, metal piping

THE DENTAL CONTRIBUTION

There can be no discussion of heavy-metal toxicity without a special reference made toward the contribution made by the dental professional in adversely impacting on human health and disease.

In 1970, an American dentist by the name of Hal Huggins published his initial findings of the harm to human function due to mercury exposure of dental amalgam fillings. In subsequent investigation, additional revelations of the potential for harm and toxicity as a result of root canals and dental extractions were also brought to public awareness. Dr. Huggins was rewarded for his efforts by having his license to practice dentistry taken away from him in an attempt to silence his powerful and unavoidable conclusions.

At this point, the public has gotten the message loud and clear concerning the health consequences of dental care. They understand that dental amalgam is a mixture that contains, by definition, at least 51 percent mercury combined with silver, tin, and copper.

From the moment the amalgam is placed in the prepared tooth, that mercury leaches out of the filling and into the mouth where it will be mixed with saliva, swallowed, and distributed throughout the body. The largest amount of leached mercury travels through a three-millimeter plate of bone that comprises the roof of the mouth where it is able to gain exposure to the brain and other neurological structures, including the eye.

Once the mercury is taken up by those tissues, it continues to accumulate and disturbs the normal function of whatever tissue is involved. The mercury is not coming out of that tissue unless extraordinary measures are taken for that purpose, which will be explained shortly.

Most everyone who reads of the horrors of dental intervention usually has a discussion with their dentist concerning the use of amalgam for dental fillings. The majority of the dentists I speak to no longer attempt to defend the use of dental amalgams as a safe material used in filling teeth. To do so with a straight face would push the boundaries of common sense. Instead, the dentist immediately changes the conversation to the use of composite materials that do not carry with them the health hazards of amalgam.

Even though the dentists do not usually attempt to make the case on how safe mercury amalgam fillings are, their professional organizations act quite differently. The ADA (American Dental Association) insists that, although mercury is a deadly element, once it is mixed by the dentist in his office and placed into the prepared tooth, the health risks of the mercury content of amalgam no longer exist.

It is tough to defend that position if you stop to consider this possible scenario. If the dentist, after mixing the amalgam on the preparation tray, should accidentally drop that mixture on the floor instead of making it to your mouth, he is not permitted to wipe the mess up with a rag. Federal and state agencies are in uniform agreement that that act has met the definition of a hazardous spill. The dentist is duty-bound to report the spill, which can only be disposed of by a HAZMAT team dispatched to clean up the mess while wearing little white spacesuits.

WHAT YOU SHOULD DO ABOUT YOUR DENTAL ISSUES

Mercury introduced into the body is never considered nontoxic. Whether or not you are knowingly ill from the exposure, you will ultimately pay a clinical price when the mercury burden has reached toxic levels. The following is a checklist of precautions for you to consider when constructing a plan to correct dental toxicity.

1. There are three things dentists can do to maintain "good dental health." The three things are

    ▫ fill decayed teeth;

    ▫ extract teeth; and

    ▫ perform root canals.

    All three of them have a health consequence, even when they are done "by the book."

    Correcting and replacing mercury amalgam fillings may be at the top of your list of things to do, but keep in mind that the other two issues have equally important health considerations. Allow me to refer you to the two books written by Dr. Huggins to appreciate a full discussion on each from the man who ought to know: *It's All in Your Head* and *Uninformed Consent*.

2. Your dentist, even if he might want to be helpful in this current health climate, is not the right professional for the job. I find most dentists all too eager to volunteer to remove all the mercury amalgam fillings and replace them with composite materials.

    To consent to the help may be a tragic decision on your part due to the fact that he is not trained in how to protect you during the amalgam-removal process. On that day, you will be exposed to the most amount of mercury that you have been on any single day of your entire life. That quantity of mercury and the "off gases" of mercury vapor have the potential to make most people ill, but some have been so devastated from the intervention that they never really recover from the experience.

    Find a "biological dentist" in your area who has been trained to use the "Huggins protocol." This is an elaborate set of conditions and equipment designed by Dr. Huggins to protect you during the amalgam-removal process. Check out the members of the IAOMT (International Academy of Oral Medicine and Toxicology).

3. Do not forget that you have three potential dental-related health issues:

   - amalgam
   - previous extractions
   - root canals

   An IAOMT-trained dentist can have a discussion with you concerning all three areas of concern.

4. After your dental issues have been resolved, you have, in a sense, only corrected the reservoir of continuous mercury leaching into the body. You will then require the assistance of a medical doctor who is trained in the correction of heavy-metal toxicity. As was discussed earlier, your current doctor will not be familiar with anything other than acute toxic poisoning.

   To locate a doctor near you, I suggest you explore two different physician organizations that train doctors in removing chronic toxic heavy metals.

   - The American College for the Advancement of Medicine: www.ACAM.org
   - The International College of Integrative Medicine: www.ICIMED.com

DETERMINING THE TOXIC BURDEN

For our purposes, it should be assumed that metals have accumulated over a lifetime and are deeply embedded in the body tissue. They will not be detected by blood testing, which in a previous discussion pretty much eliminated any help coming from your conventionally trained doctor.

Depending on the practitioner and his scope of practice, various methods of detection and quantification are possible. The patients who are seeking guidance from health professionals are usually open to discussion concerning heavy metals. They usually have a multiyear history of physical complaints and have already decided they will have to journey outside of conventional medicine if any answer has the possibility to be forthcoming.

We will discuss multiple options available for correcting heavy metals with their advantages and disadvantages. We will also discuss the means by which we can quantify the amount of the metal that is identified.

With some exception, it is anticipated that two things will occur in sync with one another. The first is that the heavy metal will be gradually eliminated from the body. The second is that the confusing symptoms that were interfering with your daily function will finally come to an end.

Hair Analysis

Hair is excretory tissue as opposed to functioning tissue. When it is analyzed and compared with symptoms experienced by a patient, it can be very helpful in confirming the diagnosis of heavy-metal toxicity. As hair grows from a follicle, elements in the body that require elimination are incorporated into it to facilitate the body in getting rid of whatever it may have in excess.

DOCTOR'S DATA: TOXIC HEAVY METALS, HAIR ANALYSIS			
	RESULT µg/g	REFERENCE INTERVAL	PERCENTILE 68th 95th
Arsenic (As)	0.021	< 0.14	
Lead (Pb)	0.38	< 3.0	
Mercury (Hg)	0.21	< 3.0	
Cadmium (Cd)	0.032	< 0.20	
Chromium (Cr)	0.52	< 0.85	
Beryllium (Be)	< 0.01	< 0.050	
Cobalt (Co)	0.010	< 0.15	
Nickel (Ni)	0.54	< 1.0	
Zinc (Zn)	170	< 300	
Copper (Cu)	160	< 70	
Thorium (Th)	< 0.001	< 0.005	
Thallium (Tl)	< 0.0001	< 0.005	
Barium (Ba)	1.3	< 8.0	
Cesium (Cs)	< 0.002	<0.010	
Manganese (Mn)	0.19	<1.5	
Selenium (Se)	0.70	<2.1	
Bismuth (Bi)	0.018	< 5.0	
Vanadium (V)	0.049	< 0.20	
Silver (Ag)	0.86	< 1.6	
Antimony (Sb)	< 0.01	< 0.12	
Palladium (Pd)	0.011	< 0.015	
Aluminum (Al)	24	< 19	
Platinum (Pt)	< 0.003	< 0.010	
Tungsten (W)	< 0.001	< 0.015	
Tin (Sn)	0.38	< 1.0	
Uranium (U)	0.26	< 0.20	
Gold (Au)	0.082	< 0.50	
Tellurium (Te)	< 0.05	< 0.050	
Germanium (Ge)	0.029	< 0.045	
Titanium (Ti)	0.70	< 2.0	
Gadolinium (Gd)	<0.001	< 0.008	

A sample toxic-element profile of hair from Doctor's Data is included here with barcode graphs depicting the levels of each of the top toxic metals that were detected.

Toxic elements may be two hundred to three hundred times more highly concentrated in hair than in blood or urine. It is for this reason that hair is the tissue of choice for the detection of recent exposure to the toxic element and is also recognized by the Center for Disease Control (CDC). The CDC also acknowledges the value of hair mercury level as a maternal and infant marker for exposure to neurologic methylmercury from fish.

It should be pointed out that hair as an exposed body appendage is vulnerable to external contamination and can be affected by shampoos, dyes, and hair treatments. It is for this reason that the recognized first step in interpreting the report is to make certain that external sources of contamination have been eliminated.

For all of the reasons previously mentioned, hair analysis should never be considered as a "stand alone" diagnostic test for heavy-metal toxicity. It requires that the information obtained from hair analysis should be interpreted in conjunction with a patient's symptoms and other laboratory tests.

Provocative Urinalysis

Acute metal poisoning is a rare phenomenon. Should such an acute phenomenon occur, blood and hair analysis are the two best ways to accurately assess the metal burden of a patient.

When discussing chronic metal toxicity, the gold standard in medicine has continued to be provocative urine testing. Due to the fact that this form of toxicity is due to exposure spread out over many years, all the toxic substances are bound up into the very matrix of cells of the body and are not available to be detected until they are initially prodded out of the cell first to be able to gain access into the blood. Once in the blood, the kidneys will remove them as they do all waste products, and then they exit the body during urination.

The provocation agents that are used are a number of pharmaceutical metal detoxification agents such as EDTA, DMSA, or DMPS. These different compounds are administered via IV or orally. The urine is collected for either six or twenty-four hours after the provocation, and a representative specimen is sent to the lab for analysis.

DOCTOR'S DATA: URINE TOXIC METALS			
	RESULT µg/g	REFERENCE INTERVAL	WITHIN REFERENCE / OUTSIDE REFERENCE
Aluminum (Al)	210	< 35	
Antimony (Sb)	0.5	< 0.4	
Arsenic (As)	40	< 117	
Barium (Ba)	11	< 7	
Beryllium (Be)	< dl	< 1	
Bismuth (Bi)	0.2	< 15	
Cadmium (Cd)	2.2	< 1	
Cesium (Cs)	8.9	< 10	
Gadolinium (Gd)	0.4	< 0.4	
Lead (Pb)	31	< 2	
Mercury (Hg)	15	< 4	
Nickel (Ni)	22	< 12	
Palladium (Pd)	< dl	< 0.3	
Platinum (Pt)	< dl	< 1	
Tellurium (Te)	< dl	< 0.8	
Thallium (Tl)	0.4	< 0.5	
Thorium (Th)	< dl	< 0.03	
Tin (Sn)	1.9	< 10	
Tungsten (W)	1.2	< 0.4	
Uranium (U)	0.2	< 0.04	

You will notice that the bar graph used to indicate the result of each metal uses the designation of either "within reference" or "outside reference." Patients often interpret the "within reference" range as normal and the "outside reference" range as not. There is no normal range for any of the toxic metals listed.

What the reference range indicates is that in every hundred people who take the test and are healthy, their urine reflects the level of toxic agents prior to disease ever taking a foothold. As those levels rise with time, they will more than likely be requesting the test with a different motivation in mind.

Fecal Metals

The administration of pharmaceutical binding agents, as we have just discussed, results in the excretion of toxic metals through the kidneys. After these results are analyzed, IV and oral chelating agents are suggested to finally reach a point when the toxic substance can be removed entirely.

The body's natural way of detoxifying heavy metals does not use this pathway. The normal detoxification pathway for the body is through the gastrointestinal system. The body's own natural detoxifier is known as glutathione, which forms a complex with the toxic metals that are excreted in the bile and pass out of the body via the feces. If you want to find out how well your natural heavy-metal detoxification is working, you analyze the heavy metals found in the feces.

Selecting the form of testing for heavy metals is not an accidental pursuit. The types of testing that are chosen all yield heavy metals. The form of testing is as diagnostic as the heavy-metal yield that is revealed. Consult with your doctor in developing the type of testing that will be ordered and know what detoxification pathway is being assessed.

REMOVING A HEAVY-METAL BURDEN

Accumulated heavy metals over decades play a prominent role in the final expression of many diseases. The majority of the eye disorders of advancing age are clearly a representative of that group. Once these heavy metals gain access to the body, the detoxification mechanism of the effective region of the body springs into action to remove them.

The primary component of that mechanism is a naturally occurring intracellular antioxidant known as glutathione, which complexes with the metal so the body can eliminate it. When heavy-metal exposure is minimal, glutathione is able to meet the demands for forming complexes and can be expected to clear the body of the offensive metal completely.

With chronic and continuous exposure, the likelihood that this outcome should be expected is very slim. You can expect that the source of exposure of heavy metals will remain steady and that the total body burden, if nothing special is done, will continue to increase. It is for this reason that a plan to provide additional measures to reverse your toxicity is mandatory.

In this section, we will describe numerous methods of reversing your heavy-metal burden. There are multiple exit routes by which heavy metals are eliminated, and the body is able to be involved in more than one at any given time. We will also discuss the advantages and disadvantages of each of them. Some will require sophisticated medical guidance while others will not. We begin this discussion with the introduction of the concept under which all forms of metal detoxification are described. That term is known as "chelation."

What is Chelation?

Chelation is a medical procedure that includes the administration of a recognized chelating agent to remove heavy metals from the body. Conventional medicine reserves their use for acute toxicity situations only, which are at best rare. The clinicians in alternative medicine appreciate their benefit to be used in cases of chronic heavy-metal toxicity over an extended period of time.

Before beginning a treatment program with these agents, some initial testing must first be conducted to reveal what metals are being retained by the body and in what quantity. Chelators are then selected based on the metals detected and their affinity to chemically bond with the chelating substance. For instance, EDTA (ethylenediaminetetraacetic acid) has its greatest attraction to bond with lead (Pb). If heavy-metal testing demonstrates a high lead toxic burden, it then becomes the agent of choice to be used for its elimination from the body. Similarly, other agents are selected when the offensive metal reveals similar affinities for other agents.

The root of administration may also be a consideration in selecting a chelating agent. There are IV, oral, IM, and rectal forms of most of the agents. Doctors trained in their use will take these factors into account when formulating their treatment plans.

Still another consideration is the chelating agent's ability to gain entrance into the "target" tissue so that it can do the job for which it is intended. By far, the so-called "blood-brain barrier" remains the biggest impediment to clearing toxic metals from the brain, and only a very limited number of agents can be selected for that purpose.

THE TYPES OF CHELATION

A good rule for you to follow is to find a doctor in your area who is trained in the diagnosis and treatment of chronic heavy-metal toxicity. You more than likely have symptoms and/or diseases that are directly related to your toxic burden and need professional help and guidance for this aspect of your treatment. The professional organizations of ACAM and ICIM who train doctors to do chelation safely and effectively are only a phone call away.

Food-Based Chelation

Although your doctor should construct your chelation program, your diet can provide assistance to it by eating foods known to be able to remove heavy metals. With this in mind, these foods should be added to the diet. They are collectively referred to as natural heavy-metal chelators.

1. Amino acids: As a bonus to meat eaters, proteins found in many products are made up of so-called building blocks known as amino acids. They are found in abundance in other foods like eggs and fish. They work to increase liver function and balance enzyme production.

2. Cilantro: A super herb that can effectively remove heavy metals (specifically aluminum, lead, and mercury), cilantro is also known as an immune booster.

3. Onions and garlic: The sulfur in these two foods can also eliminate heavy metals. Other foods with high sulfur content are items like cauliflower, Brussels sprouts, and cabbage.

4. Brazil nuts: These nuts are not necessarily able to eliminate heavy metals but work to restore minerals like selenium and zinc that may be depleted during the chelation process.

5. Chlorella: This is a mild chelating helper.

6. Food-grade activated charcoal: Dr. Al Sears recommends twenty grams per day of the food-grade form of activated charcoal for both general detoxification and detoxing heavy metals. The twenty grams should be spread out in two to four doses in a twelve-hour period over a twelve-day span of time.

Pharmaceutical-Based Chelation

This form of chelation can be traced back to the early 1930s when a German chemist, Ferdinand Munz, was first to synthesize EDTA as a replacement for citric acid as a water softener. Chelation therapy itself began in World War II when it was learned that it could be effective in treating lead poisoning. Since its introduction in the United States in the 1950s, many doctors developed sophisticated protocols and rules to follow to use these chelators efficiently and safely. Other chelating agents have also been studied and can be employed by these trained professionals with equal confidence.

The following is the list of pharmaceutical chelating agents:

- EDTA
    - the first of all chelating agents
    - effective in the removal of lead, arsenic, cadmium, iron, and copper
    - can be administered via IV, orally, or rectally
    - the most frequently used of all chelating agents
- DMSA
    - approved for the removal of lead in children
    - primarily administered orally
    - the only one of all chelating agents that can cross the blood-brain barrier to remove lead and mercury
- DMPS
    - used as the most-effective agent in mercury heavy-metal toxicity
    - primarily administered via IV but also available in oral form
- Alpha-lipoic acid
    - a very good heavy-metal chelating agent
    - able to cross the blood-brain barrier
    - is effective for removal of mercury

- increases body levels of glutathione

Pharmaceutical-based heavy-metal detoxification is effective, but it will take time for the heavy-metal burden to be alleviated. Strict monitoring of the patients will be required over this time period to ensure that the heavy metals being eliminated do not overload the elimination mechanisms of the body. A close watch of kidney function is imperative since it is the site where the heavy metals ultimately are eliminated from the body. Consulting with trained chelation doctors will be your greatest ally in this endeavor.

Glutathione-Based Heavy-Metal Detoxification

The body's own natural elimination of metals is dependent upon complexes formed between a metal and a naturally occurring intracellular detoxification substance known as glutathione. The availability of glutathione in quantities sufficient enough to accomplish this task will determine how effective the body can be in dealing with toxic heavy metals. If the heavy-metal contamination is sustained or if glutathione activity is compromised, the consequences of metal toxicity can be expressed if there is not a way to provide an elevated amount of glutathione to accomplish this task.

Dr. Patricia Kane, a world-renowned PhD in biochemistry, has been the leader in developing protocols to deal with correcting disease that adversely affects cell metabolism. Her now-famous P-K Protocol demonstrated the ability to remove heavy metals and to do so without the use of pharmaceutical chelators. Instead, Dr. Kane advocates the use of administering IV or oral glutathione in quantities that allow complexes to form with heavy metals and those complexes to be eliminated by their natural route via the gastrointestinal system.

She has trained a number of doctors in the United States who can perform her protocols. Inquiries can be made as to their locations at the office of BodyBio located in Millville, New Jersey, to identify a physician in your area with this training.

Natural Chelation

A relatively new approach to removing heavy metals has been introduced by Edward Kane, CEO of BodyBio, which accomplishes that task as the second step of a two-step process.

In Step 1, a "taste-testing" technique is used to determine deficiencies of eight macrominerals required by the body. Those minerals include:

potassium	copper	molybdenum
zinc	chromium	selenium
magnesium	manganese	iodine

Once the deficient minerals are determined, a daily supplementation regime is continued until a repeat "taste test" confirms that the mineral deficiency has been corrected.

Step 2 relies on the fact that the replaced minerals end up displacing heavy metals that reside within the cell membrane, mobilizing them to enter the tissue fluid. Once in the tissue fluid, they can complex with glutathione and be eliminated from the body naturally.

In a sense, you get two for the price of one. First, you replace the much-needed macrominerals for normal functioning of the body. Second, replacing the minerals allows you to mobilize heavy metals and have those metals removed by the body's natural glutathione-elimination mechanism.

CHAPTER 8

OPTIMIZE PERFUSION

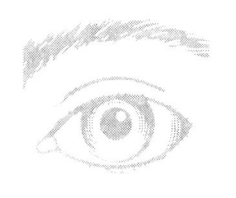

Earlier in this book, I described in great detail the three components required to return tissue to full function by providing a vehicle by which nutrients can be delivered to a cell and waste products can be taken away. The large arteries themselves, those blood vessels that bring nutrients to a cell, are not usually compromised sufficiently to limit the amount of blood that arrives into the region of the cells. It is, however, the network of capillaries that permits the final delivery to occur.

These microscopic blood vessels have a semipermeable membrane which consists of small openings for oxygen and other nutrients to pass out of the arterial system into the tissue fluid and, from that medium, enter the individual cells. The entire system of these microscopic arteries and veins (venous capillaries) is collectively referred to as the microvasculature. It is within these vessels that life cannot only be merely sustained but optimized.

It has been amazing to me that our friends the cardiologists who spend so much time and effort to reestablish blood flow of the large arteries through the invasive means of catheterizations and stent placements literally ignore the opportunity to amplify the microvasculature. It is probably to my advantage that by not having the training or experience to perform catheterizations or place stents that I have concentrated on the microvasculature as the target for optimizing blood flow to the tissues. It may not be as "sexy" as performing a cath, but in terms of optimizing blood flow to the tissues, it has no equal.

There are four modalities that will allow you to optimize the microcirculation to the cells of the body. To emphasize that point, let me further clarify that I am referring to every "nook and cranny" of human tissue that will function better with reestablishing optimal blood flow to that area, and the eye is no exception.

The retina of the back of the eye rarely, if ever, loses the delivery of blood to it by the large arteries. On the other hand, the microvasculature of the retina with advancing age always has some limitation to blood flow as these blood vessels literally "dry up" over time. Combine that with the diseases of the retina that lead to damage of whatever blood vessels remain, and you have the formula for having not just impairment in your vision but losses that will progressively worsen over time.

As we now begin to discuss how to optimize blood flow to all parts of the body, let's revisit a few facts on how you arrived here and how you will become better. Up until this point, you should be aware of the following:

1. Your eye disease is a combination of three factors that have led you to develop your eye disorder. These three factors are

    - nutrient deficiencies that you have accrued over a lifetime;

    - the accumulation of toxic substances and the very matrix of the cells of the eye equally over a lifetime; and

    - the final blow is the inability to adequately perfuse the tissues of the eye, which bring the first two into play and ensure that your eye disease will remain unresolvable until perfusion has been restored.

2. The structures of the eye that are not working properly can be revived to full function once again if these three conditions are corrected.

3. Because your eye doctor is not trained to think that your vision can be restored, he frequently insists "nothing can be done."

4. The Three-Step Program to regain your sight consists of numerous activities aimed at correcting the cause of your vision loss. These activities can be done on your own at home or as a part of an aggressive three-day program.

For those who are interested in maximum improvement, in a short period of time I will complete the introductory portion of this chapter with the following statement of fact: "Eight-five to ninety percent of the patients who participate in the office-based program will have a substantial improvement in their vision in three days."

THE FOUR MODALITIES TO OPTIMIZE PERFUSION

Modality 1: External Counter Pulsation (ECP)

With a more sedentary lifestyle and advancing age, your microvasculature is eroding with each passing day. It is accurate to say that we achieve our maximum number of capillaries in our later teenage years or early adulthood. For those who continue to pursue cardiovascular challenges through such activities as long-distance running or cycling, that maximum level of microvasculature is extended considerably.

With the sole exception of progressive cardiovascular disease leading to the occlusion of blood vessels due to plaque deposition, your number of arteries and veins remain stable throughout your lifetime. When you finally depart this good earth, you end up leaving with the same number of these large vessels that you entered with as a child.

It is the microvasculature that does not withstand our movement through time. Theoretically, when you wake up tomorrow, your network of microscopic capillaries will be less than you took to bed with you the night before. What this means is that your ability to deliver nutrients to your cells and to take waste products away from them progressively worsens over time. This phenomenon is the explanation for all diseases of advancing age.

If we just focus on the eye alone, it becomes abundantly clear why such diseases as glaucoma and macular degeneration, with rare exception, are not found in the twenty- and thirty-year-old populations. In those unfortunate, much younger individuals that do suffer from retinal disease, it is actually their genetic predisposition which leads to accelerated disease processes in the eye.

With the exception of this small group of individuals, the eye diseases that have been mentioned are found only in individuals of advancing age, and the final escort that brings them to full expression is the loss of the microvasculature in the retina and other regions of the eye.

If this disease process is to be reversed, it will only be possible as a result of restoring the microvasculature to optimal function once again. Take all of the supplements that you want. Pursue detoxification as aggressively as humanly possible to no avail. The fact of the matter is that you will not be successful, because your transit system for delivering those nutrients and removing toxic waste is not available to carry out the task.

Once again, let the message be clear that the ravages of age and diminished blood flow can be reversed. It is possible to return your capillary network to function once again. The first measure that we will discuss that will accomplish this is a medical modality known as ECP.

ECP (external counter pulsation) was created in the 1980s and is an FDA-approved and potentially insurance-covered procedure. As potent a force as ECP is, it is very difficult to find. There are clinicians throughout the country that do offer it. Although you more than likely will not be fortunate to find it available in your backyard, you will most certainly find it in your region. We will address the availability of ECP a little further on in this section. For the moment, let's discuss what ECP does and how it does it.

ECP is the only modality I am familiar with that can actually develop a brand-spanking-new set of blood vessels that you do not even own right now. Just think about that for a moment. Even though the devastation of time has "dried up" your microvasculature in your retina, you can get it back. You will not have to take a drug or any pharmaceutical preparation. Even though vigorous exercise is beneficial, you will not need to join a health club or obtain the services of an athletic trainer.

The oldest patient I have ever treated with ECP was ninety-four years old. He did need some assistance to get onto the device, but once in position, he did not need to twitch a single muscle to receive the full benefit of the treatment. This fact has been extremely helpful in treating an elderly population where other diseases have advanced to such an extent that ambulation is severely compromised.

What Does an ECP Treatment Consist Of?

Let me draw your attention to a photograph of an ECP device with a patient in position to initiate a treatment. As you can see, the patient is lying in a comfortable position. She has large inflatable cuffs around her extremities, one set around each of the calves, another

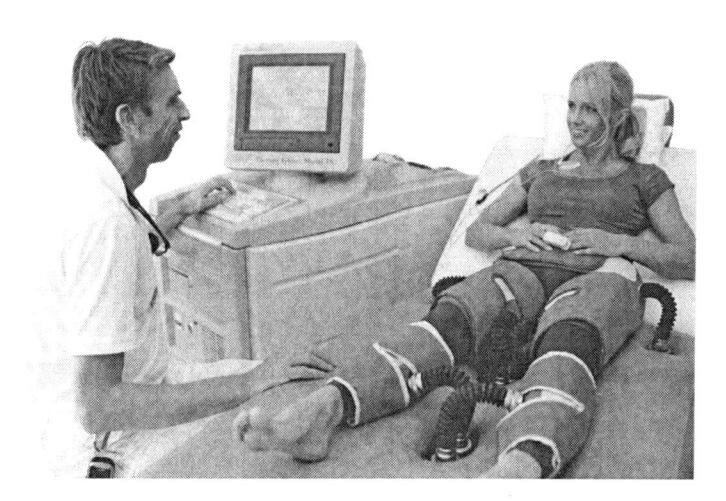

ECP

set around each of the thighs, and an additional cuff placed around the buttocks and pelvis.

The cuffs have a similar construction to a blood-pressure cuff in that there is an inflatable bladder in each of them. When the bladder is inflated with air, the cuffs immediately constrict the legs and pelvis in a similar fashion as would occur with taking a blood pressure.

The difference is that the size of the tubing that propels the air into the cuff is not like the small rubber hose of a blood-pressure device. Instead, it is a large-caliber corrugated hose. The other big difference is that, instead of a squeezable rubber bulb to blow up the cuffs incrementally, they are filled by a very large compressor found under the bed. When the compressor fires, there is an immediate and forceful squeeze around the extremities and the pelvis.

The second component of an ECP bed is that the control panel acts as an EKG (electrocardiogram) device. Three small leads are placed on the chest, which allows the device to accurately display your own heart rhythm. At that point, the device knows where you are with each heartbeat. It knows if the heart is contracting or relaxing or anything in between.

Once the two main components of the ECP device are in place (the cuffs and the EKG), it is time to turn the switch on to have the ECP device cycle rhythmically and in synchronicity with the contraction of the heart.

During the contraction phase of the heart (systole), the cuffs are deflated. The compressor fires at the precise point in the heart cycle that the heart begins its relaxation phase (diastole). The first cuffs to fill are those that are around the calves. Fifty milliseconds later, the cuffs around the thighs are filled and constrict. Fifty milliseconds after that, the same thing occurs with the cuffs around the pelvis. When you add up all of your 50 millisecond intervals, you then determine that all of the cuffs have been filled in just over one-tenth of a second. At that point, the heart enters another contraction phase of the heart cycle, and the cuffs are deflated once again. This means that if you have a heart rate of seventy-two beats per minute, the ECP device cycles seventy-two times in synchronicity to it.

The entire treatment lasts one hour. I know that your first reaction may be that you are not sure you can tolerate an ECP treatment for an hour. Let me share with you that I understand that initial apprehension. Let me also share with you that when I peek into the ECP room in my office, what I observe in the vast majority of patients is that they are sleeping quite comfortably through the ECP treatment. My own first ECP treatment had me feeling equally concerned. All I can tell you is that within five minutes of the start of your first treatment, you will realize, as do others, that an ECP treatment is actually quite pleasurable. I swear, quite pleasurable.

What Does an ECP Treatment Do?

Now that I have fully described what you may have incorrectly perceived as the agony of an ECP treatment, let me take this time to explain what undoubtedly is the ecstasy of it. My initial statement about ECP bears remembrance. ECP is the only modality that will allow you to both create a new and, at the same time, restore a previously functioning microvasculature that has been diminished with age. It is for this reason that I encourage all of my patients to consider incorporating ECP into their treatment program no matter what their particular health challenge may be. It then only stands to reason that it should be included as part of your efforts to regain your sight.

So that I can clear up how ECP can accomplish the restoration of your microvasculature, let's discuss the physiology of what is happening in the body during an ECP treatment.

If you recall, your legs and pelvis are being squeezed in sync with your natural heart cycle. Keep in mind that when the cuffs are inflated, that inflation occurs first in the calves, then the thighs, and then the hips. That type of squeezing order results in all your blood volume below the waist being forced above your waist at each ECP cycle. When the cuffs deflate, all the blood returns back to the lower portion of the body only to be forced above the waist at the next ECP cycle.

Greater than 50 percent of your total blood volume is found below the waist. That 50 percent is being forced above that line with every cycle of the ECP device. This volume of blood has never been seen by the arterial system in the upper part of the body before and can only be made to do so with mechanical intervention. Nevertheless, every ECP cycle is delivering that enormous volume of blood to all of the arteries and, consequently, all of the body parts above the waist, including the eye.

The first thing to mention is even though the volume of blood delivered to all these tissues is considerable, it is *not* harmful in any way. What needs to be appreciated is that the arteries receiving that quantity of blood have a hormonal mechanism to try to accommodate it. Even though they never will really accomplish the accommodation, they still have a mechanism available to try.

You see, blood vessels secrete a very special hormone when exposed to these large volumes of blood. The hormone is called "VEGF." VEGF stands for vascular endothelial growth factor. That hormone is rarely, if ever, secreted by the arteries because there is never such a significant volume of blood that requires urgent accommodation. The ECP device provides that urgency. The arteries secrete the hormone VEGF, which under its influence causes new blood vessels to grow instantaneously. That is correct. You grow a brand-new set of blood vessels around every party of the body that secretes it, including the eye.

Let's be clear. Under the influence of VEGF, you do not grow any new arteries. That number remains constant. What you do grow, and plenty of them, are those microscopic blood vessels that were referred to as the microvasculature. It is through ECP that we can begin to supply the body tissue with the nutrients that just could not get there before. You have just taken a step to undo what the passage of time has created. You can now have the three-step equation working for you to achieve what the aging process has taken away—a functioning microvasculature network.

ECP Considerations

To make the discussion of ECP more complete, we should take the time to present some additional related issues regarding ECP. The medical doctors who run ECP facilities in your area will be aware of these items, but in an attempt to make you an enlightened consumer, let me try to tackle a few of them for you.

1. **AAA**. If you qualify to do ECP, you should know that this procedure is completely safe and cannot harm you in any way. There are some contraindications to ECP. The first of these is absolute, meaning that ECP is never permitted to be done in a group of patients who have evidence of an abdominal aortic aneurism, or so-called triple A.

    Some individuals have a defect in their aorta, which is the largest artery in the body by which all of the arteries branch from. This aneurism is an outpouching or dilatation of the aorta with a diseased or weakened wall, which allows it to grow in size to such a degree that it actually can rupture. If that should happen, the mortality associated with such an event is greater than 95 percent, even with the immediate availability of surgical intervention.

    It is a mystery to me as to why it is never routinely checked for, but in fact it is not. Any facility that offers ECP will check for it by ordering an abdominal sonogram. If a triple A is detected, ECP is contraindicated because of the potential for an abrupt rise in blood volume within it, which will cause it to grow even larger or possibly rupture.

    If a sonogram does not detect the presence of a triple A, you should be assured that no such event is possible. In my fifteen years of doing

ECP, I have encountered four patients with a triple A. The number of patients I have assessed is now well into the thousands.

Those four patients were not permitted to do ECP. Three of the four went on to have it surgically repaired. One had his triple A monitored and never did have surgery. Remember, if you do not have a triple A, you are not going to develop one, yet each candidate who wishes to do ECP will be checked. The protocol doctors follow is clear. If there is a triple A, there can be no ECP.

2. **Relative contraindications for ECP**. The presence of a triple A is an absolute contraindication. There are a couple of relative contraindications that should also be mentioned that are much more common. Relative contraindications mean that maybe you can do ECP or maybe not.

   The first of these is a condition known as aortic regurgitation, which is a leaky valve on the left side of the heart. In this anomaly, blood passing through a valve at the origination of the aorta flows backward because the valve does not fully close.

   This can be visualized on an echocardiogram of the heart. It has four classifications. Grade 1 and 2 usually can do ECP and receive the full benefit from it. Grade 3 occasionally can also do ECP. Grade 4 is severe enough that ECP is contraindicated, and the patient more than likely is a candidate for valve replacement surgery.

3. **Pleasurable experience**. As I have said, ECP is a pleasurable experience. The majority of patients having an ECP treatment fall asleep. Some patients, however, have rapid heart rates due to some heart anomaly. In these situations, ECP is not pleasurable but is downright uncomfortable. Rather than listing the disorders, let's just say that your doctor will treat you for each to have your heart rate in a

safe and controlled range that will make ECP the enjoyable experience that it should be.

4. **Referral**. You need a referral to do ECP. That referral can only come from a cardiologist. They control ECP in that the insurance company will only reimburse for the procedure with the accompanying referral.

   It always has amazed me that so few cardiologists actually do ECP in their offices. They are far more interested in the "sexy" procedures like catheterizations and stent placement. When you do find a facility that does ECP, it will either be operated by a cardiologist or at least work closely with one. They make the final decision as to whether or not you qualify for a referral to do ECP.

5. **Length of ECP treatment**. ECP is usually done one hour a day, five days a week, for seven weeks. It has been determined through research that at around thirty-five treatments, optimization of the benefits of ECP should be achieved.

   For those patients who travel a considerable distance, the ECP protocol, which is honored by insurance companies, does allow for two ECP treatments a day. The only qualification concerning the two-treatment protocol is that there must be at least one hour that separates Treatment 1 from Treatment 2. In this way, patients will be required to be at the facility for at least three hours a day in order to compress the time from seven weeks to three and a half weeks. This is greatly appreciated by someone who may travel two hours to the facility or who has come from out of town to participate in our ECP program.

6. **Insurance coverage**. ECP is not a "one-and-done" experience. The insurer will reimburse for this treatment annually as long as it is accompanied by the corresponding referral from a cardiologist. I can

only deduce that the insurer feels that the benefits to a patient are so plentiful that they must feel they are receiving a good return on their investment. In that same way, they are not really happy with the big stuff.

Invasive procedures such as catheterizations, stent placement, and coronary artery bypass grafting (CABG) are not good returns on investment. The cost of them is astronomical when compared to ECP. The results are not long lasting. Stents are sometimes re-occluded in a week and need to be repeated. Bypass grafting of the coronary arteries, when done with veins harvested from the legs, have an average life expectancy of seven years.

ECP done annually can usually allow patients to avoid either of the two medical interventions. By the time one year has elapsed since your last ECP round was concluded, you would always benefit from another round of this microscopic revascularization procedure. At about the ten-month mark, if our patients have not already contacted us for their annual cardiovascular workup, we call them. In that way, they never really are able to creep back into poor levels of perfusion to any body part, including the eye.

Modality 2: The BEMER

ECP was presented as the modality that allows the participant to develop new blood vessels in the microvasculature that did not exist previously. These minute blood vessels that form the microvasculature network do not just suddenly "dry up" and go away. That evolutionary process is a slow one and occurs gradually over the course of many years to decades. The cells that depend on nutrients supplied to them by this network of blood vessels are literally starved to death or, said in a more accurate way, "starved to dysfunction and disease."

A vigorous exercise regimen could easily resolve the diminished blood flow to slow this starvation phenomenon. However, human nature and degenerative disease being what they are, with advancing age it is more commonly associated with a decrease in vigorous physical activity and in its place the adoption of a sedentary lifestyle.

The stage is then set and will be played out with the anticipated conclusion. At a time when we need "naturally generated" blood flow to the microvasculature, we receive even less volume of blood to the tissues, and the vicious cycle to perpetuate disease becomes established. Is there anything we can do to turn this around? The answer to this question leads us to the discussion that describes the three remaining modalities that, although not being able to develop new blood vessels as was the case with ECP, can still optimize the blood flow to the microvasculature in both the newly acquired and previously established microscopic blood vessels.

The first of the remaining three modalities is a representative and outgrowth of the well-established science of quantum physics. You do not have to be able to completely understand such a complex scientific domain to be able to appreciate how we can use quantum physics for a medical benefit. There are only two concepts that require explanation. One will be presented here and another in the discussion of the next modality. We begin with Concept 1, EMF, or electromagnetic field.

In the quantum world, everything has its own unique signature, electromagnetic field. That means everything. Whether it is alive or dead, natural or man-made, all things have their own EMF.

Of course, the human body has its own EMF, but it goes even further than that. It is not just the body that emits a unique EMF. It is that each tissue of the body has its own specific, signature EMF. A nose, for instance, has its own EMF. A kidney has its own unique EMF. Yes, the eye has its own EMF too.

This is why an MRI (magnetic resonance imaging), the most sophisticated radiographic study available in today's medical world, can give us such sharp and clear pictures of the inside of the human body. The different organs have their own unique EMF set up, distinct lines of demarcation where an organ is clearly visible, and the organ right next to it with another EMF is also sharply defined. The pictures that result are as sharp and well-defined as any high-definition photograph. The whole thing is as a result of how medical science has applied the knowledge acquired through the use of quantum physics.

BEMER

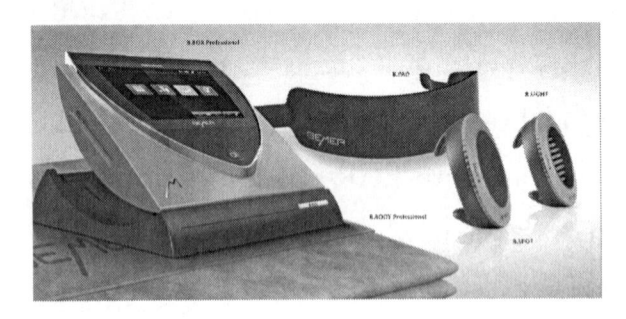

With that same concept in mind, it is time to introduce you to a newer medical contribution to harness EMF. This new technology is a member of a group of devices known as PEMF (pulsed electromagnetic field). The device is a contribution made by a German scientist, and it is known by the acronym BEMER (bio-electromagnetic energy regulation).

As you can easily see here, the BEMER consists of a console and a cloth mat. Inside the mat are multiple coils that emit an EMF that is not continuous but pulsed. You either sit or lie on the mat, and the entire body is penetrated by the EMF emitted by the coils. I should mention that while receiving a BEMER treatment, you have no awareness or perception of that EMF exposure. It is a completely innocuous experience.

The BEMER emits only one EMF, and it happens to be a rather important one. The EMF emitted by the device is specific for blood vessels. When the body is exposed to the signature field for blood vessels, there is a physiological response that occurs whereby blood flow is augmented considerably that is known as "vasomotion." This incredible "boost" in blood flow to vasomotion results in optimal blood flow being generated into the microvasculature within six minutes, and after the completed eight-minute treatment has concluded, the increase in blood flow is sustained for up to sixteen hours.

The BEMER is a great complement to your ability to restore your lost vision. It provides the greatly increased blood flow to all body tissues, including the eye. It works on any of the microvasculature that you currently possess. What makes perfectly good sense to me is to first complete a round of thirty-five treatments of ECP. As a result, you will develop a new microvasculature that did not exist before you started. Once you have completed your ECP program, taking a "daily ride" on the BEMER will maintain your newly acquired microvasculature while you resurrect your old one.

It is not practical or safe to have an ECP unit in your own home. It is every bit of both of those to have your own BEMER. The company, although located in Lichtenstein, Germany, has a wide sales network in the United States, Canada, and other parts of the world. To find out more, visit www.BEMERAmerica.com.

The BEMER is beneficial in restoring many tissues of the body back to full function once again. It can be used by any family member no matter the age or disease. It only makes sense that an optimal blood flow to diseased tissue will improve function over time. The BEMER has the distinct uniqueness to be used by every member of the family and for any condition, whether that may be acute or chronic.

Modality 3: FSM (Frequency-Specific Microcurrent)

In the next discussion, we return to the quantum world to provide a benefit not appreciated by conventional medicine. The first quantum concept that provided for the discovery of the BEMER was the fact that all things, living or dead, have their own unique EMF. To describe the next modality, it is necessary to explain a second quantum concept.

Quantum Concept 2 is that all matter has its own vibratory signature that is unique to it and only it. This vibratory rate is quantifiable and is known as frequency. Every single bit of matter is vibrating at a specific, unique, and signature frequency.

In keeping with our explanation of EMF and the examples found within the human body, the tissue of the nose vibrates at its own unique frequency. A kidney cell vibrates at its own frequency. The eye, of course, does too. It goes even further than that because the eye has many parts, each with a unique function. Consequently, each of those parts has its own vibratory or frequency also. Knowing what those frequencies are is obviously important in optimizing blood flow, but the full use of that knowledge requires an in-depth explanation because, with that explanation, so much more is possible than the treatment of blood flow alone.

Electrical Stimulation: The First Medical Use of Current

Forty years ago, the use of electroceuticals emerged in Western medicine with the advent of units referred to as either electrical stimulation or TENS units (transcutaneous electrical nerve stimulation). These units remain popular to this very day and have gained that popularity by virtue of their ability to alleviate pain.

Electrical stim is provided by leads that are attached to the skin on one end while connecting to the battery-powered current-producing device at the other end. The idea is to gradually turn up the voltage of the current (voltage is the force that supplies the current) to a point that you can actually feel the current being delivered to the body. You are supposed to bring up the voltage where it feels uncomfortable and then back off the intensity until it is easily tolerated.

Let's use an example of someone with right knee pain secondary to surgery. The knee hurts for obvious reasons. The person just had surgery, so it is easy to say it hurts because it is supposed to hurt and then gradually diminish as the tissue heals. The reason the person perceives the pain is only due to the sensory nerve impulses that are sent by the knee to the brain. The pain response is only possible because the brain is receiving input coming from the knee.

The current of an electrical stimulation device is delivered to the body at a dose measured in milliamperes, which means thousandths of an ampere. This is a mammoth amount of electrical current for the body to accommodate. It is such a large amount of electrical current that it completely "jumbles up" the sensory message that is being sent by the knee to the brain. As a result, that message never arrives. The pain that the patient is experiencing is appreciated only if the message arrives there, so in a very real sense there is no pain to be experienced.

TENS UNIT

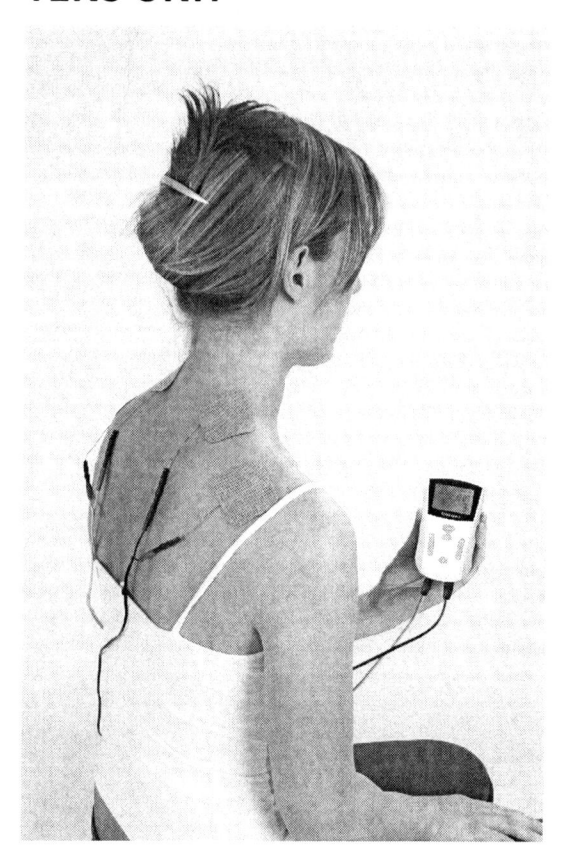

You can see why these devices became so popular. People wore them all day every day. They became ingenious on how to conceal them so that aesthetically they could receive pain relief, and nobody would even know.

Although not harmful in any way when the person finally shut off the device, nothing really changed either. Tissues remained inflamed, pain returned, and the person reapplied the device the next day. If the pain was due to an arthritic knee, there have been patients who have worn a TENS unit or electrical stim machine for thirty years or more. The development of electroceuticals needed to take a giant leap so that a sustained benefit could be possible. That leap came in the 1990s and is called FSM.

The Next Leap: FSM (Frequency Specific Microcurrent)

Electrical activity is how we as living beings function. There is a constant moving of electrical energy but certainly not in the magnitude of a TENS unit. The energy of the device was in an overpowering amount of thousandths of an ampere (milliampere).

In a very real sense, it should be called "macrocurrent" or "mammoth current." A refinement needed to be made to step the current down to those amounts in harmony with the body. The next leap in the development of microcurrent came in the late 1980s as the result of the monumental and pioneering work of Charles McWilliams, MD. Dr. McWilliams, an original student of the German electro acupuncturist Dr. Reinhold Voll, used his understanding of electrical current to develop groups of frequencies that could elicit predictable responses in the body to achieve an anticipated outcome. His frequencies serve as the basis for all microcurrent used by clinicians today. It is for that reason that he has been recognized as the "godfather" of modern day frequency specific microcurrent. He and his wife Susan continue to maintain a large medical practice on the island of Nevis in the Caribbean.

Microcurrent is measured in millionths of an ampere, which is the level of naturally flowing electrical current in the body. Delivering electrical current at that level is in complete sync and harmony of all physiological processes within the body.

THE BLUE BOX

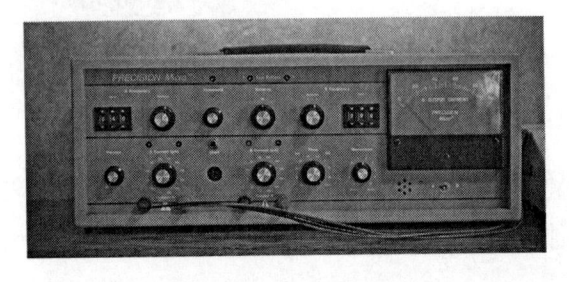

The first microcurrent devices that were available for medical use weighed over sixty pounds and were referred to as "the blue box." It did allow for a very special medical benefit in that it permitted one to select the frequency of the current that was put into the body.

It was as a result of that discovery that microcurrent made a giant leap. Medical science owes a great deal of gratitude to the contributions made by Dr. Carolyn McMakin who constructed a device that permitted not only the input of the microcurrent in millionths of an amp but was able to deliver that current as a frequency pair. One of the frequencies was targeted at a specific selected tissue while the other was targeted to a specific selected pathology. The device was miniaturized to make it portable.

Dr. McMakin also developed the first courses that could be offered to teach others how to do the same, and the study of FSM was well on its way to becoming what it is today.

How Does FSM Work?

We can finally return to how this section on microcurrent began in those initial two quantum concepts.

Concept 1: All tissue has its own unique EMF signature.

Concept 2: All tissue has its own unique frequency signature.

MACULA

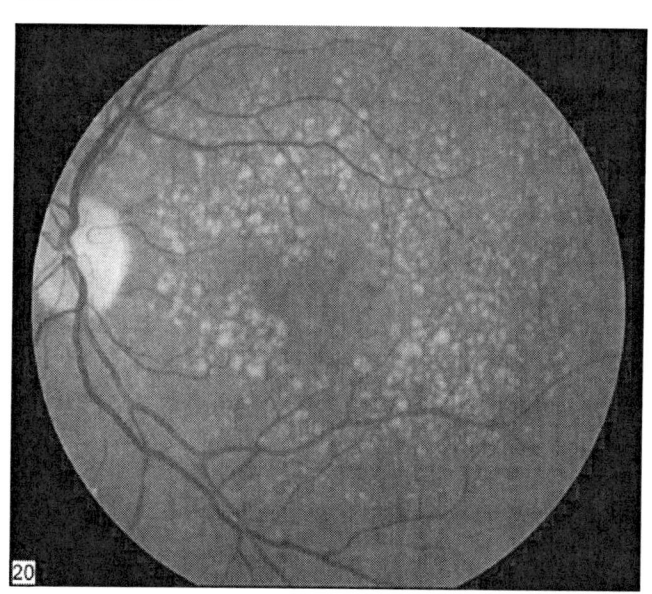

These are not only concepts, but they are also constants in that they do not ever change. What has changed is being able to use them both for medical benefit, and you can finally be the recipient of the benefit of that knowledge.

You are now in a position to appreciate why it is that the Three-Step Program relies so heavily on the use of FSM.

I know that our initial discussion dealt with how to optimize blood flow. I hope that I have not confused you, but it is now time to reveal how FSM can correct everything, including blood flow, so let's return to our example of the eye once again.

The eye has multiple parts, each performing a specific function. For the purpose of being accurate, I have chosen to discuss a very important part of the retina known as the macula. It is found essentially in the center of the retina. Remember, I could have picked any part of the eye.

According to the medical literature, it is known that a healthy macula of the eye vibrates at 137 Hz (Hertz). What can be said is if someone has a problem with the macula, macular degeneration for instance, that macula is not going to be vibrating at 137 Hz.

When the FSM device is programmed to supply current into the body, it can specifically program that current to vibrate at a frequency of 137 Hz. In so doing, I can immediately and profoundly make that macula resonate or vibrate at the 137 Hz level.

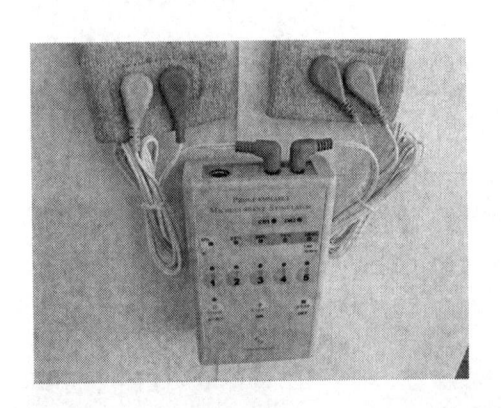

An analogy that helps to explain this is the vibrations that occur when striking a tuning fork on a hard surface. For example purposes, we will choose a C-note tuning fork. While it is vibrating at an auditory C note, if I take another C-note tuning fork and strike it onto a hard surface, it now too resonates at an auditory C note. When both tips of these two tuning forks are allowed to touch, the C-note vibratory activity is increased in strength of the auditory C note that is heard. The reason is that the two are in harmony and in sync with one another. The only thing that can result is the sound of a healthy and crisp C note.

Returning to the previous description of the macula allows for a better understanding of how FSM works. Putting microcurrent into the body at a frequency of 137 Hz can only target one part of the body that vibrates at that frequency—the macula of the eye. It will make the diseased macula which is not vibrating at a frequency of 137 Hz resume that healthy and innate frequency once again.

Once the FSM program is complete, it does not mean the macula will stay vibrating at that level. For that to happen, we will need the other member of the frequency pair—the frequency to reverse the pathology.

When we program FSM devices, we always program the current as frequency pairs. One of the pairs is determined to be the healthy frequency of the body part we are trying to correct. The second member of the frequency pair is meant to combat a pathology, which is affecting the normal functioning of that body part.

Just as every body part has its own frequency, every pathology also has its own frequency or vibratory rate. In the case of a diseased macula, there may be many pathological forces preventing the macula from vibrating at its healthy rate of 137 Hz.

One common pathology to most tissue is inflammation. It is a large player in most disease and certainly could be a reason why the macula is not resonating at its healthy frequency. I do not know what frequency inflammation vibrates at. Honestly, I do not want to know. What I do know is that a frequency of 40 Hz stops inflammation immediately. What makes good sense is that when I program the frequency pair for the macula, one of my frequencies will be 40 Hz (to cancel out inflammation) and the other at 137 Hz (to have the macula vibrate at a healthy level again).

We usually use the phrase "the issue with the tissue" to keep in mind that when the device is programmed, we should select the pathology cancellation frequency first and then select the frequency of a target tissue that we want to bring back to health. A full program may contain ten to fifty pairs. It may take anywhere from fifteen minutes to two hours to run an entire program. Some programs can be so long that they are done during sleep because they may last up to six hours.

This section has provided me with the opportunity to explain the contribution made by FSM in the treatment of eye disease as well as many others. It truly is the workhorse of the three-step, three-day program as well as an anchor as a home modality.

The issue of microcurrent would not be complete without a special mention made to a giant in the realm of electroceutical therapy, Dr. Jerry Tennant. Dr. Tennant, an illustrious eye surgeon and ophthalmologist, devised and then created a microcurrent device he named appropriately the "Biomodulator." His invention is not frequency specific but instead delivers microcurrent at a higher voltage to facilitate healing and to replace diseased tissue.

His now-famous text on the subject entitled "Healing Is Voltage" is a must-read for clinicians and laypersons alike. He literally had to invent a treatment to correct his own health challenges when conventional medicine told him that "nothing could be done." His superior intellect allowed him to become a pioneer in the development of microcurrent devices. We frequently use his creation in our eye program. I cherish my relationship with Dr. Tennant and consider him both a colleague and a friend.

FSM: This All Started with Blood Flow

Every body part can have an FSM program written for it. Our discussion began with how to optimize blood flow to your eye. FSM has numerous frequency pairs that can be programmed to reverse all eye disease. As you may have already surmised, FSM also has a capability to do much more than optimize blood flow alone. It is a key component to the success of the three-step and three-day programs to restore your vision. You want to be certain that you have a frequency specific microcurrent machine with programs written specifically for your eye disease. Many pathologies can be addressed, but one constant to all those programs is to optimize perfusion.

Precautions with FSM

I want you to be certain of your success after completing this book. With those best of intentions, let me take the time to point out a couple of items to you at this particular time. Having just completed the discussion on microcurrent, every element of the Three-Step Program can be done by you at home with local medical talent.

The one element that will require sophisticated participation by a medical doctor will be the proper programming of a frequency specific medical device. It even goes much further than that. When it comes to diseases of the eye, that assistance can only be through the help of an ophthalmologist who is trained in the programming of an FSM device.

As a nonophthalmologist medical doctor, I feel completely comfortable writing FSM programs for most medical conditions and diseases. What I have set as a rule for myself is that when it comes to diseases of the eye, the device needs to be programmed by an ophthalmologist who is trained to do it.

I have heard many horror stories by patients who were impressed by the power of FSM in cognitive disease who were persuaded by nonmedical or ancillary medical personnel who claimed to have the knowledge of the frequencies to program an FSM device. In a best-case scenario, the patient just did not become any better. At worst, these patients had their disease accelerated.

Dr. Edward Kondrot did not discover FSM, but he was the first ophthalmologist to use FSM to correct eye diseases. The success of his now-famous

Three-Day Program, which I follow without alteration, gives testimony to that fact. He has modified the program only slightly over the twelve years that he has offered it. The results have been astounding and have allowed me to state numerous times: "Eight-five to ninety percent of those patients who participate in the program will have a substantial improvement in their vision in three days."

If the Three-Day Program is not convenient for you at this time, you may want to participate in a two-day program where the objective is to have a microcurrent device programmed for you by Dr. Kondrot. You do not need to be seen by Dr. Kondrot in order for him to be able to program the device; you only need to send your medical records to him from your ophthalmologist that you have maintained throughout the course of your medical management.

Modality 4: Nutraceutical Development of the Microvasculature

In the study of medicine, it is not uncommon to have something learned in the treatment of one disorder to have a crossover impact in a completely unrelated treatment of another. This adage describes what we have learned from the podiatric community in their confrontation with the late-stage consequences of diabetes.

An all-too-frequent complication in this disease is the decrease in blood flow to the small blood vessels in the lower extremities as a result of an occluded microvasculature. In these patients, the blood flow to the feet is so compromised that even the tiniest wound can result in gangrene to the toes and forefoot because of extremely poor circulation to the feet. All that it takes is a small wound produced by careless toenail clipping to start a cascade of events that ultimately culminates in an amputation of the foot to spare the life of the patient.

It is the domain of podiatry to deal with the medical problems that can occur from the ankle down to the toes. It is for this reason that the diabetic population can be expected to have the phone numbers of their podiatrist of choice to receive early foot care in an attempt to avoid a tragic loss of limb. We thank these specialists for helping to prove that a combination of vitamins has shown the ability to either prevent or even reverse these peripheral vascular complications in the diabetic population.

Metanx is the name of a prescription form of vitamins B6, B12, and folic acid that over an eight- to twelve-week program can establish the regrowth of blood vessels to replace the diseased tissue of the foot and toes of these individuals and prevent the cascade of gangrene from moving forward to amputation. These outcomes have been widely published in the medical literature and have prompted many medical doctors to treat their diabetic patients proactively far in advance of the first symptoms of such peripheral vascular disease.

Metanx is different in a number of ways when compared to over-the-counter forms of the three vitamins that are contained in it. These are the differences:

1. The amounts of each vitamin contained in a tablet are as follows: folic acid, 2.8 milligrams; vitamin B6, 25 milligrams; vitamin B12, 2 milligrams

2. The folic acid is found in its biologically active form of L-methylfolate. Over 50 percent of the general population cannot convert folic acid to L-methylfolate, and it may be for this reason that patients have vascular disease to begin with.

3. The FDA has determined that the most folic acid that is allowed to be sold in an over-the-counter (OTC) form of folic acid is one milligram or less. The usual OTC dose is four hundred micrograms. There is a prescription form of L-methylfolate approved by the FDA, known as Metanx. It contains four times the amount of the OTC brands.

4. The L-methylfolate of Metanx is much better absorbed by the lining of the intestines when compared to folic acid.

The daily dose of Metanx is two tablets a day. It will take approximately three months to have major regrowth of the microvasculature. Once you have completed a three-month protocol of the two-tablet-per-day regimen, you should continue staying on Metanx for the long haul to maintain the microvasculature that you have created.

It should be reiterated that there is nothing available in the medical literature to confirm this microvasculature benefit in the foot as occurring in the eye with equal success. Most clinicians agree that we should be able to expect similar results no matter what the disease, no matter what the area of the body that is involved. Fifty percent of the population cannot convert folic acid to its active form of L-methylfolate. It seems quite probable that the genetically acquired condition must be considered when treating any disease, especially the eye.

CHAPTER 9

GETTING BACK TO KEEPING IT SIMPLE

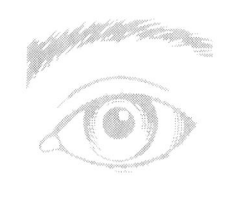

It has been my intention to present a simplified Three-Step Program to restore your lost vision. For the sake of being complete in my explanation of the three steps, I may have lost you by this point in this book because you are probably thinking the program is not as simple as you thought it was going to be. Let me assure you that even though the detailed description of the program may appear onerous and daunting, it still remains only three steps to accomplish your objective to regain your sight.

To assist you in reestablishing your comfort level with the simplicity of the Three-Step Program, I have written this chapter. Part 1 is referred to as the "CliffsNotes version" of the book where each chapter is reduced to the most significant details only. You may elect to either read the entire first eight chapters and then use Chapter 9 as a quick reference guide or just read Chapter 9 alone. Having these options allows you to decide how to start. If you are a detail-oriented learner, the details are provided. If you like to cut through "the thick" of the details and find the bare facts only, permit me to assist you in that endeavor.

It is not my intention to have the book be placed on a shelf of your bookcase. It is to be used as a workbook and guide to regain your vision. Do not allow yourself to become bogged down in the minutiae of detail. Those details are in the book when you require clarification only. In those instances, they will allow a more elaborate explanation of the concept in question. This book is a Three-Step Program to regain your sight. Start your program to receive the vision improvements you seek.

In Part 2 of this chapter, it is my intention to further demonstrate the simplicity of the Three-Step Program. In this section, I have included a "matchbook-cover" version of the book. That is right. This book can and will be reduced to fit on one side of a matchbook cover. Every meaningful detail of this book can be reduced to this micronized version and still provide you with the only reference that will be required to start the Three-Step Program.

Every Three-Step Program I conduct has this "matchbook-cover" version presented to the participants multiple times over the three days. I frequently refer to it as a "pop quiz," and I will spring it on them without warning throughout the three-day experience. By the time they leave, they have received the message loud and clear. They are not confused. They are ready to take on their eye disorder and win.

The program is and has always been three steps:

1. Correct deficiencies.

2. Remove toxicities.

3. Optimize perfusion.

THE THREE-STEP PROGRAM TO REGAIN YOUR SIGHT PART 1: THE "CLIFFSNOTES VERSION"

Chapter 1: Where We Are

- The frequently used description of your disease as "nothing can be done" that has been said by your doctor is a fallacy.

- Do not allow anyone, especially your eye doctor, to tell you "nothing can be done."

- Your eye doctor does not have the tools or training to restore your lost vision. From his perspective, "nothing can be done" is accurate. From our perspective, it is not.

Chapter 2: Can This Program Work for Me?

- Disorders of the cornea can best be treated by conventional medicine.

- Disorders of the retina are correctable through integrative medicine (see complete list of disorders on pages 4 and 5).

- Surgical intervention should always be a "last resort."

- Retinal injections should always be a "last resort."

Chapter 3: The Retinal Diseases

- Wet macular degeneration deserves special consideration because of injections into the back of the eye used to stop bleeding.

- These anti-VEGF injections should always be a last resort only due to an 18.3 percent chance of producing global atrophy at the injection site.

- You must develop a "fair-shake plan" to allow you to avoid these injections.

- Glaucoma and the elevated intraocular pressures associated with this disorder must be brought under control.

- Eye drops prescribed by your eye doctor should never be discontinued or decreased by any other doctor.

- Diabetic retinopathy can also demonstrate retinal bleeding. Injecting them should also be a "last resort."

Chapter 4: Let's Take a Step Backward for a Moment

- Medical doctors are trained to combat disease.

- Conventional medicine uses a combination of surgery, procedures, and drugs in fighting disease.

- You can never fight a disease and win. The forces of the disease are much too powerful to overcome.

- Integrative doctors are trained in promoting health. You can promote health and win.

Chapter 5: The Plan: A Three-Step Program to Regain Your Sight

- KISS: Keep It Simple, Stupid.

- There are only three steps to regain your sight.

- These three steps will not just correct your vision problem, but they are also the formula for correcting all diseases of advancing age.

- You cannot win by trying to combat a disease. This is the error of conventional medicine.

- You can win if you restore health. This is the reason alternative medicine works.

Step 1: Correct all deficiencies.

- You cannot eat your way to health because there are no longer enough nutrients found in the soils so that your food source can provide them to you.

Step 2: Remove all toxicities.

- Toxic substances accumulated in the tissues will not allow them to function properly.

- The medical profession only recognizes acute toxicity. Your toxic burden is chronic. Because of this, you have just hit a brick wall and will not be able to receive any help from your doctor.

- If you want to identify heavy metals, you must analyze the urine, not the blood.

Step 3: Optimize perfusion.

- Blood flow is the medium by which nutrients arrive and waste products are taken away from a cell.

- If there is no blood flow, you cannot ever correct deficiencies or remove toxicities.

- Step 3 is the most overlooked step of the three by conventional and alternative medicine doctors alike.

Chapter 6: The Three-Step Program to Regain Your Sight

Remember, you will not be able to eat your way to health.

Rule 1: You can take your current diet and, by eating organic, remove the harmful components to your fresh food choices.

Rule 2: Avoid GMOs.

- Genetically modified organisms (GMO) have an altered DNA within the food and have created a "franken" molecule in the process.

Rule 3: You do not have to avoid meat.

- Select free-roaming, grass-fed, grain-free, antibiotic-free animal products.
- Fats are good, and you need a lot of them.
- Eat certified organic livestock or their local equivalent.

Rule 4: Shop the periphery of your supermarket.

The center of the store has all the processed foods. Stay away from the center.

- The periphery has the perishables. Make sure you buy organic. Stay away from the ten most common food additives.

Rule 5: Eat nutritive-dense carbohydrates and avoid the starches.

Rule 6: Of the three foods (proteins, fats, and carbohydrate), by far the most important are the fats.

- You have to replace seventy trillion cells every ninety days.
- Your fat consumption assures the body that it has the raw materials to complete that task.
- There are six components of optimal supplementation:

    1. A good multivitamin

    2. Adequate macro minerals

3. Adequate micro minerals

4. Appropriate fatty acids

5. Enzymes for proper digestion and assimilation

6. Antioxidant protection

- There is a formula for sensible supplementation.

Chapter 7: Removing Your Toxicities

- Inevitably, the accumulation of toxic substances will prevent tissue from normal functioning.

- Your eye disease has been at least partially provoked by this toxic burden.

- It is possible to identify and quantify your toxic-metal burden.

- Although many metals can be involved, the most frequently identified heavy metals are the following:

  - mercury
  - lead
  - cadmium
  - aluminum

- Dental intervention is plagued with contributing to toxicity by

  - amalgam fillings;
  - root canals; and
  - tooth extractions.

- Only allow a biological dentist to correct dental toxicities.

- The most accurate testing to determine heavy-metal burden is provocative urinalysis.

- There are pharmaceutical and natural chelators that can remove all toxic metals.

Chapter 8: Optimize Perfusion

- Of all the steps in the Three-Step Program, by far the most important of the three is to optimize perfusion.

- The blood is the medium by which nutrients are delivered to a cell and waste products are taken away. The greater the volume of blood, the better the cells will be able to function as a result of this delivery and removal process.

- The most important way to increase blood delivery to the cells is through the microscopic blood vessels known collectively as the microvasculature.

- There are four ways to optimize perfusion:

  1. ECP (external counter pulsation)

     - An FDA-approved and potentially insurance-covered modality is able to develop a new microvasculature in every organ in the body, including the eye.

     - A round of ECP consists of thirty-five treatments, which are administered one hour a day, five days a week, for seven weeks.

     - It is permitted by the insurer to be done once a year.

CHAPTER 9: GETTING BACK TO KEEPING IT SIMPLE

- Find it in your area.

2. The BEMER: A PEMF (pulsed electromagnetic field) device

- Every tissue has its own unique signature electromagnetic field (EMF).

- This device produces the EMF specific for blood vessels and, as a result, greatly increases blood flow to the microvasculature.

- One eight-minute treatment is all that is required to optimize blood flow in the microvasculature and then maintain that level of blood flow for sixteen hours.

3. FSM: frequency specific microcurrent

- Every tissue of the body also has its own unique, signature vibration that is referred to as frequency.

- FSM devices can be programmed to cause tissues of the eye to vibrate or resonate to their healthy frequency while at the same time cancel out the pathologies that provoke the diseases of the eye.

- The frequencies that can be programmed into the device optimize blood flow to the microvasculature of the eye.

- All participants in the Three-Step Program should have an FSM device programmed for their specific eye disease by a qualified and specially trained ophthalmologist.

4. Nutraceutical formation of the microvasculature

- There are a large number of individuals (greater than 50 percent of the general population) that cannot convert folic acid to its active form known as L-methylfolate.

- Patients with microvasculature disease have demonstrated the ability to revascularize body tissue by taking daily supplements containing large amounts of L-methylfolate over a twelve-week period.

- Metanx is a prescription form of vitamin B12, B6, and folic acid in the form of L-methylfolate. Patients should take one tablet twice a day.

THE THREE-STEP PROGRAM TO REGAIN YOUR SIGHT PART 2: THE "MATCHBOOK-COVER" VERSION

Step 1: Correct all deficiencies.

- organic diet
- sensible supplementation

Step 2: Remove all toxicities.

- pharmaceutical chelation
- nonpharmaceutical chelation
    - foods based
    - glutathione based
    - "natural" chelation

Step 3: Optimize perfusion.

- ECP: external counter pulsation
- PEMF: the BEMER
- FSM: frequency specific microcurrent
- nutraceutical

CHAPTER 10

WHERE DO WE GO FROM HERE?

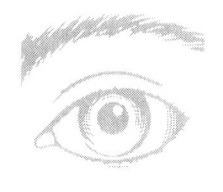

At this point, the journey I describe in the opening pages of this book is nearly complete. You are now prepared to assume the control of your destiny in reestablishing your vision. The Three-Step Program and its component parts have been demystified. You can see yourself achieving the successful conclusion that you were told could never occur.

You think differently now. You will not permit naysayers to dampen your enthusiasm to regain your sight. They will have to come to grips with their ignorance by the results of your efforts and the improvements in your ability to see. Do not become consumed by the misinformation they have provided you. At this stage in your development, that would truly be a misuse of both your time and energy.

Your mission is to take your newly acquired knowledge and direct your attention to follow the Three-Step Program as it now has been thoroughly explained. There is too much riding on the improper use of your time. A few additional insights will assist you in putting your plan in play.

IDENTIFY LOCAL TALENT TO ASSIST YOU IN CARRYING OUT THE THREE-STEP PROGRAM

There are many professionals who possess the skill set to assist you in correcting deficiencies and removing toxicities. Whether that help is available through chiropractic, naturopathy, osteopathy, or allopathy, you should shop around for a "good fit" between yourself and those that you select to be on your team.

The team members you select do not have to remain static. You have to "feel right" about your team. When you do not, move quickly in making a roster change that engenders the harmony you are seeking. As your vision improves, you will find that your criteria for determining who will be best to help you will also improve. The guiding principle to all your efforts remains to maintain a focus on improving your vision and not permit negativity from anyone who claims to support your ultimate achievement or vision restoration.

IDENTIFY AN INTEGRATIVE MEDICAL DOCTOR TO ASSIST YOU

I do appreciate how difficult it can be to find a local physician who is trained in nonconventional approaches in treating disease. Difficult, yes. Impossible, no. Every region of the United States has a small group of integrative doctors that may not have a medical practice across the street but more than likely can be found across town.

I recommend using the resources of the two largest alternative medical-doctor groups in the country that maintain a database of their membership that can inform you of the closest physician to your location simply by entering your zip code at their website in their physician-identifier section. These are the two organizations:

- The American College for the Advancement of Medicine: www.ACAM.org

- The International College of Integrative Medicine: www.ICIMED.com

These integrative doctors can provide the entry point to allow you to unlock the entrance into the scientific world of organized medicine.

There are always lab tests and medical studies that will provide you with objective and quantifiable assessments of your progress. Keeping track of your toxic-metal burden through laboratory testing is the aspect of your Three-Step Program that will continue to be monitored over time. This laboratory analysis requires a prescription provided by a licensed medical doctor. Be positioned to enjoy the benefits of a symbiotic relationship with organized medicine while at the same time maintaining a safe distance of separation. The Three-Step Program does not require any prescription pharmaceutical preparations to achieve successful restoration of your vision. Keeping this fact in mind should be a guiding force for both you and your doctor.

1. Develop a "fair-shake plan."

To keep everybody honest and, more importantly, assure a participant that he or she will not be inappropriately encouraged to have injections or surgery, a fair-shake plan should be constructed. In such a plan, your medical eye doctor's recommendation that you may require an invasive procedure should be verified by an optometrist who is also monitoring your status.

The optometrist, who is not trained to do invasive procedures, has no bias in his assessment of you to do the invasive procedure or not. If he sees that your condition is worsening, he will tell you to have the procedure done. If he sees that your condition is stable, or even improving, he can advise you that you do not need the procedure.

All invasive procedures have the possibility to provoke unintended consequences. To make certain that your eye condition meets the criteria to accept the risk of an invasive eye procedure, a fair-shake plan provides you with an additional layer of protection.

2. Utilize FSM—the miracle maker for vision restoration.

You have frequently read throughout this book a statistical fact that has emerged over fifteen years of doing three-day eye programs: "Eighty-five to ninety percent of those who participate in the program will have a substantial improvement in their vision in three days."

Even though multiple modalities are used by the participants during the three days, one modality stands out as the champion in producing the outstanding results that have been experienced. Frequency specific microcurrent (FSM) is that champion that we rely on to give our participants a giant boost to start their journey to restore their lost vision.

As you now prepare to do the same, you will want to plan to include FSM as a high-priority item on your checklist of things to do. Remember, FSM devices are programmed for you and you alone. In the Three-Day Program I have been associated with, only Dr. Edward Kondrot, a board certified ophthalmologist and creator of the three-day protocol, programs each device to the specific eye disease of each patient. As a result, it is accurate to say that the device is both frequency specific and patient specific.

If there is to be a starting point for you to restore your lost vision in any capacity other than the Three-Day Program, you should make FSM that starting point. By using FSM at home, you will benefit from vision improvements as though you are a full participant. You may decide to do a Three-Day Program at some future date but be able to enjoy the vision improvements during that time lag. FSM is the true "miracle maker" and workhorse of the Three-Day Program. Make it your workhorse too.

3. **Make it all happen: optimize perfusion.**

The final step of the Three-Step Program will bring about the success of the first two steps. You have been given four different ways to optimize perfusion. Each of these individually is a powerful contributor to increasing blood flow to all body tissue. Collectively, the circulatory forces of augmented blood reach parts of the body that have not seen that amount of blood volume in thirty to forty years, or even longer. By virtue of such an increase in flow, tissue function can be restored to levels that cannot be achieved in any other way. Your vision as well as many other body functions will improve as a result of this optimization process. Make it a high-priority item on your to-do list.

STEM CELLS: THE NEXT MILESTONE IN VISION RESTORATION

It has been an overwhelming experience for me to be able to assist the vision impaired in regaining their sight. As a new group of patients leave the clinic upon completion of a Three-Day Program, their facial expressions cannot conceal the joy they are experiencing. They realize they can recapture that which they believed they had lost forever. The end of the program actually turns out to be the beginning of a long-lasting relationship that continues for many years.

During each subsequent visit with them, a looming question invariably is introduced into the conversation. "I am happy with my progress," they say, "and I continue to do the daily protocol I was originally taught, but is there anything else I can do to speed up the process?" Patients universally want to do better and do it faster. It does appear that our answer of slow and steady may be ready to be changed. Stem cells have now become a reality, and a breakthrough appears to be on its way.

It is still too premature to statistically present how successful stem cells will be, but all indications are that when they are combined with the Three-Step Program, the next big boost to vision restoration is finally in play. At the appropriate time, the results of stem cell infusion will be described and published, but all preliminary data point to a need to revise our response to the question, "Is there something else I can do to speed up my progress?"

What is appropriate at this time is to begin the process of making you a better consumer of stem cells. You need to be skilled in how to ask the right questions about how to identify the appropriate kind of stem cells that will produce the results you are looking for. Let's begin that dialogue. There are only a few concepts that will need to be explained to make you an expert consumer and allow you to make correct decisions about stem cell therapy.

Dr. Kondrot has always had a keen interest in the use of stem cells in treating eye disease. A number of years ago, he visited the experts who were using stem cells in Europe, particularly multiple clinics in Germany. These pioneers in the stem cell world spoke highly about how effective stem cells could be, but their results were miniscule when compared to the outcomes of the Three-Day Program he had already created. To put it mildly, he was not impressed by what he saw. Retrospectively, he can now accurately identify why those results were so poor. Let's now point out the lessons learned by Dr. Kondrot and, in the process, hone your understanding of what to look for in the stem cell selection process.

A Stem Cell Primer

There are two different kinds of stem cells. They are known as either autologous or homologous. The autologous form of stem cells comes from you and is then given back to you. This, of course, means that no concern of adverse reaction or rejection is possible because nothing foreign is going to be introduced into the body. There are generally recognized to be three sources of autologous stem cells:

1. PRP: platelet-rich plasma

2. Fat stem cells

3. Bone marrow stem cells

In all three forms of autologous stem cells a body "fluid" specimen is obtained and then centrifuged. This separates cells from plasma in all three cases. The result in by-products from the spinning are then injected back into the donor to obtain a positive response.

Platelet-rich plasma (PRP) is obtained by taking a generous blood sample from you and then placing the test tubes into a centrifuge to "spin them down." During this step of the preparation, all the cells in the specimen collect in the bottom of each tube while the clear, plasma portion, of the blood remain in the top of each tube. A clear line of demarcation is easily seen where the two components meet. This line is slightly irregular in its presentation and is known as the "buffy coat."

The plasma found just above this "buffy coat" contains a condensed suspension of growth factors that stimulate the formation of endogenous growth factors which can regenerate healthy cell components such as collagen and elastic fiber.

The other representative autologous stem cells are prepared for injection into the body in a similar manner by first centrifuging and then extracting the growth factors. It all sounds so good, but hidden in the explanation is the reason why autologous stem cells do not necessarily pack the wallop of the intended payoff. In fact, the tepid results of stem cell infusions that Dr. Kondrot observed in the German clinics were all of the autologous type.

There, of course, is a problem. You see, stem cells are only as good as the donor who donates them. Specimens taken from young donors are packed with youthful growth factors. If you are a young athlete attempting to recover from an injury, autologous stem cells provide a wonderful opportunity to fully recuperate and to do so rapidly. If you are a seventy-year-old with macular degeneration, the healing factors of the specimens that are donated have little to no vibrancy available to accomplish the task of regenerating diseased tissue.

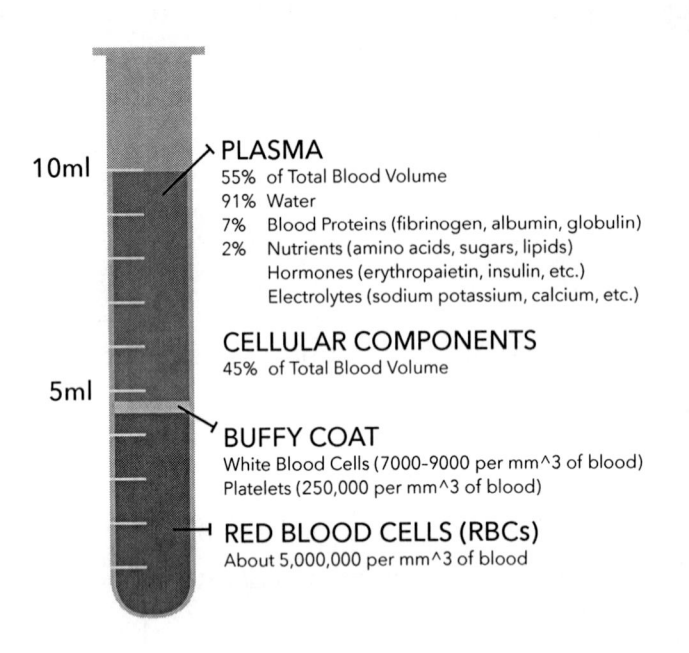

PLASMA
55% of Total Blood Volume
91% Water
7% Blood Proteins (fibrinogen, albumin, globulin)
2% Nutrients (amino acids, sugars, lipids)
Hormones (erythropaietin, insulin, etc.)
Electrolytes (sodium potassium, calcium, etc.)

CELLULAR COMPONENTS
45% of Total Blood Volume

BUFFY COAT
White Blood Cells (7000-9000 per mm^3 of blood)
Platelets (250,000 per mm^3 of blood)

RED BLOOD CELLS (RBCs)
About 5,000,000 per mm^3 of blood

In eye diseases and disorders associated with advancing age, the use of autologous stem cells does not really make sense. They may have been helpful at an earlier period in a patient's lifetime, but realistically, it is not at all common to find macular degeneration or any other retinal disease in a population of twenty-five-year-old individuals to suggest that autologous stem cells even need to be considered.

Homologous Stem Cells

We are just now entering a tremendous surge in the availability and use of homologous stem cells. Homologous stem cells come from someone else and are then given to you. They are often described as seeds that, once implanted, grow into the tissue type of whatever organ they landed in.

It is all made possible by the fact that the cells are harvested from the placenta and umbilical cord of mothers who have been screened for particular health issues and then deliver their babies by scheduled C-section. The placenta and cord are only taken after the child is born. To be honest, it would have been discarded anyway.

Cells found in these fetal tissues have not fully differentiated into any specific cell type and are said to be "multipotent." They will make the final commitment of becoming a specific cell type based on the tissue they become implanted in. If a stem cell lands in the lung, it becomes a lung cell. It is a new and vibrant lung cell to boot. If the cell lands in the kidney, it becomes a kidney cell. If the cell lands in the retina of the eye, it becomes a retinal cell. Are you beginning to see the possibilities here? The age of the patient does not really matter. It is the age of the donor that matters, and these cells are so young that they have not even determined what cell type they will ultimately become.

A second important consideration has to do with whether or not homologous stem cells can cause any reactions from the recipient's immune system. This, of course, was not a concern with autologous stem cells, because the donor and the recipient are one and the same. Homologous stem cells have been alleviated of HLA antigen during processing and are considered not to be immunologic. This means that they do not provoke any rejection reactions to the recipients immune system. This factor allows these stem cells to meet the golden rule of all good medical treatment. Stem cell therapy is both safe and efficacious.

There are three types of homologous cells:

1. Embryonic stem cells

2. Amniotic stem cells

3. Umbilical cord stem cells

From conception until two months of age, a newly formed zygote is technically referred to as an embryo and after two months as a fetus. It is illegal worldwide to obtain tissue from embryos for any medical or scientific purpose. President George Bush signed the law to make that official in the United States early in his administration. There is no need to mention it any further other than to make the discussion complete.

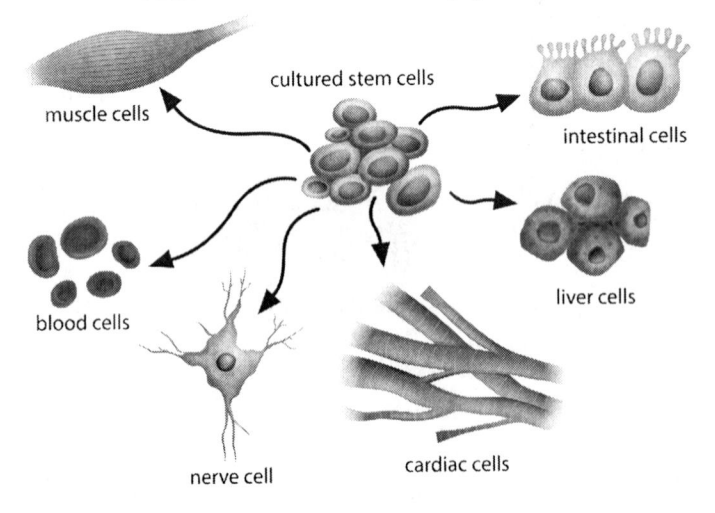

Amniotic stem cells are the mixture of cells obtained from amniotic fluid that the growing fetus is literally immersed in during pregnancy as well as cells from the amniotic membrane itself, which is a sac that surrounds the growing fetus. A certain portion of those stem cells are from an extremely important cell line referred to as mesenchymal cells that are predetermined to develop into such tissues as skin, cartilage, heart, nerves, muscles, and blood vessels. It will be from this cell lineage that the vast majority of medical possibilities will be derived to revive diseased and dysfunctional tissues of their recipients.

Umbilical cord blood collected at birth is also a rich source of stem cells that can be harvested for medical purposes. There is actually a growing trend for parents to request that cord blood specimens be collected at the birth of their child, frozen, and cryogenically stored for the future medical needs of their child. There is no reason to think this practice will do anything but become common medical practice as stem cell therapy becomes more widely accepted.

Of the two stem cell types that are currently being harvested for medical use, umbilical cord stem cells are showing the greatest promise. The reason for this is that cord blood possesses greater mesenchymal cell content than any other source of human origin, and that cell line has the greatest potential to reverse disease.

Your consumer enlightenment education of stem cell therapy is just about complete. Some final details will give you the ability to ask the right questions when anyone attempts to suggest that you should consider their stem cell product. This industry will burgeon in the next decade. Here are some of the questions that will lead you to make a correct decision based on medical fact and not emotional vulnerability.

Question 1: Are the stem cells autologous or homologous?

Autologous stem cells (PRP, fat, bone marrow) are less effective when elected as a source to treat the diseases of advancing age. They may be fine in young athletes, but their ability to reverse disease in an aging population is at best minimal. Proceed cautiously if anyone claims to be able to help reverse your eye disease through the use of autologous stem cells.

Question 2: How many stem cells do I receive with your product?

This turns out to be a very important question when determining which homologous stem cell product you should choose to have administered to you. Stem cells are juvenile and metabolically very active. They have a doubling time of approximately three to six weeks. This means that if in one milliliter or ml (the standard dose used in the industry) there are one million stem cells, three to six weeks later they will have doubled to two million cells. Three to six weeks after that, there will be four million stem cells, and so on. The progeny of the initial one million cells never really stops providing. It makes sense that the greater number of cells you start with, the greater the likelihood is that your eye disease will be improved.

The FDA has set a minimum standard that in a one-millileter vial, there must be at least thirty-two million cells. To date, there are very few companies that can meet this thirty-two million minimum and consequently do not meet the minimum standard for FDA approval of their product. Just ask the question: How many stem cells are found in one ml of your product? They have to know the answer to that question. Shop around and listen for the answer to be "at least thirty-two million."

Question 3: How often do I have to undergo stem cell therapy?

Based on the doubling rule of three to six weeks, an industry moniker is becoming universally accepted. That moniker is expressed in the phrase "one and done." Stem cell therapy should only require one treatment. Things should be just becoming better with time after that.

Remember, those cells and their progeny never stop providing. That means the benefit to you never really stops either. If you elect to repeat stem cell therapy, you can certainly do so and should expect even better results with time. There are individuals who actually do an annual "spritz" approach to stem cell therapy. Once again, that is their decision. I am just pointing out that multiple homologous stem cell treatments should not be a condition set by the facility in order to participate in the program they offer.

Question 4: Is the stem cell product heparin free and preservative free?

The FDA has set a second standard for the stem cell industry in order to meet with their approval. That standard is that the stem cell product must be preservative free. The cells are flash frozen at the time of harvest. They remain frozen until they are prepared for use. No one knows of the possible damage to stem cells due to exposure to synthetic chemicals. It seems that if the FDA does not go there, you should not either.

Your stem cell primer is now complete. You are an enlightened consumer of stem cell therapy and able to look for the answers to questions that will allow you to make appropriate decisions about your healthcare in general and your eye disease in particular.

It appears that, for a change, the FDA is out in front of the stem cell industry. Very few companies meet FDA criteria for their approval. You only need to ask, "Is your product FDA approved?" You can make your first question lead to the need to ask the second.

The stem cell industry will undergo light-years' worth of changes over the next decade. What is known today may become obsolete tomorrow. As I monitor the changes, it will become my responsibility to report back to you through some form of media of those changes. I envision the dawning of a wonderful opportunity to correct disease.

RESOURCES

CHAPTER 1:

Siahpush, Mohammad. "Postmodern values, dissatisfaction with conventional medicine and popularity of alternative therapies." *Journal of Sociology* 34.1 (1998): 58-70.

Furnham, Adrian, and Julie Forey. "The attitudes, behaviors and beliefs of patients of conventional vs. complementary (alternative) medicine." *Journal of Clinical Psychology* 50.3 (1994): 458-469.

Fontanarosa, Phil B., and George D. Lundberg. "Alternative medicine meets science." *Jama* 280.18 (1998): 1618-1619.

Egede, Leonard E., et al. "The Prevalence and Pattern of Complementary and Alternative Medicine Use in Individuals with Diabetes." *Diabetes Care* 25.2 (2002): 324-329.

Pagán, José A., and Mark V. Pauly. "Access to Conventional Medical Care and the Use of Complementary and Alternative Medicine." *Health Affairs* 24.1 (2005): 255-262.

Klassen, Terry P., Margaret L. Lawson, and David Moher. "For randomized controlled trials, the quality of reports of complementary and alternative medicine was as good as reports of conventional medicine." *Journal of Clinical Epidemiology* 58.8 (2005): 763-768.

O'Shea, Tim. *Conventional Medicine vs. Holistic: A World of Difference.* San Jose, CA: NewWest, 1999. Print.

CHAPTER 2:

Sivak-Callcott, Jennifer A., et al. "Evidence-based recommendations for the diagnosis and treatment of neovascular glaucoma." *Ophthalmology* 108.10 (2001): 1767-1776.

Rumelt, Shimon, Yosef Dorenboim, and Uri Rehany. "Aggressive systematic treatment for central retinal artery occlusion." *American Journal of Ophthalmology* 128.6 (1999): 733-738.

Scott, Ingrid U., et al. "A randomized trial comparing the efficacy and safety of intravitreal triamcinolone with standard care to treat vision loss associated with macular Edema secondary to branch retinal vein occlusion: the Standard Care vs Corticosteroid for Retinal Vein Occlusion (SCORE) study report 6." *Archives of Ophthalmology* 127.9 (2009): 1115.

Duker, Jay S., and Mark S. Blumenkranz. "Diagnosis and management of the acute retinal necrosis (ARN) syndrome." *Survey of Ophthalmology* 35.5 (1991): 327-343.

Fontanarosa, Phil B., and George D. Lundberg. "Alternative medicine meets science." *Jama* 280.18 (1998): 1618-1619.

Ni, Hanyu, Catherine Simile, and Ann M. Hardy. "Utilization of complementary and alternative medicine by United States adults: results from the 1999 national health interview survey." *Medical Care* 40.4 (2002): 353-358.

Margalit, Eyal, and Srinivas R. Sadda. "Retinal and optic nerve diseases." *Artificial Organs* 27.11 (2003): 963-974.

Duker, Jay S., and Mark S. Blumenkranz. "Diagnosis and management of the acute retinal necrosis (ARN) syndrome." *Survey of Ophthalmology* 35.5 (1991): 327-343.

CHAPTER 3:

Bird, A. C., et al. "An international classification and grading system for age-related maculopathy and age-related macular degeneration." *Survey of Ophthalmology* 39.5 (1995): 367-374.

Friedman, David S., et al. "Prevalence of age-related macular degeneration in the United States." *Archives of Ophthalmology* 122.4 (2004): 564-572.

Ferris, Frederick L., Stuart L. Fine, and Leslie Hyman. "Age-related macular degeneration and blindness due to neovascular maculopathy." *Archives of Ophthalmology* 102.11 (1984): 1640-1642.

Ferris 3rd, F. L. "Senile macular degeneration: review of epidemiologic features." *American Journal of Epidemiology* 118.2 (1983): 132-151.

Klein, Ronald, et al. "The epidemiology of age-related macular degeneration."*American Journal of Ophthalmology* 137.3 (2004): 486-495.

Hyman, Leslie G., et al. "Senile macular degeneration: a case-control study."*American Journal of Epidemiology* 118.2 (1983): 213-227.

Bressler, Neil M. "Age-related macular degeneration is the leading cause of blindness…" *Jama* 291.15 (2004): 1900-1901.

Avery, Robert L., et al. "Intravitreal bevacizumab (Avastin) for neovascular age-related macular degeneration." *Ophthalmology* 113.3 (2006): 363-372.

Orlin, Anton, et al. "Association between high-risk disease loci and response to anti-vascular endothelial growth factor treatment for wet age-related macular degeneration." *Retina* 32.1 (2012): 4-9.

Wong, Tien Y., Gerald Liew, and Paul Mitchell. "Clinical update: new treatments for age-related macular degeneration." *The Lancet* 370.9583 (2007): 204-206.

Meads, C., et al. "Clinical effectiveness and cost-utility of photodynamic therapy for wet age-related macular degeneration: a systematic review and economic evaluation." (2003).

Dixon, James A., et al. "VEGF Trap-Eye for the treatment of neovascular age-related macular degeneration." Expert opinion on investigational drugs. 18.10 (2009): 1573-1580.

Yoganathan, Pradeepa, et al. "Visual improvement following intravitreal bevacizumab (Avastin) in exudative age-related macular degeneration." *Retina* 26.9 (2006): 994-998.

Oliver-Fernandez, Alejandro, et al. "Progression of visual loss and time between initial assessment and treatment of wet age-related macular degeneration." *Canadian Journal of Ophthalmology/Journal Canadien d'Ophtalmologie* 40.3 (2005): 313-319.

Oliver-Fernandez, Alejandro, et al. "Progression of visual loss and time between initial assessment and treatment of wet age-related macular degeneration." *Canadian Journal of Ophthalmology/Journal Canadien d'Ophtalmologie* 40.3 (2005): 313-319.

Kulkarni, Amol D., and Baruch D. Kuppermann. "Wet age-related macular degeneration." *Advanced drug delivery reviews* 57.14 (2005): 1994-2009.

Joussen, Antonia M., and Norbert Bornfeld. "The treatment of wet age-related macular degeneration." *Dtsch Arztebl Int* 65 (2009): 3.

Garba, Adinoyi O., and Shaker A. Mousa. "Bevasiranib for the treatment of wet, age-related macular degeneration." *Ophthalmology and Eye Diseases* 2 (2010): 75.

Arias, Luis, et al. "A study comparing two protocols of treatment with intravitreal bevacizumab (Avastin) for neovascular age-related macular degeneration." *British Journal of Ophthalmology* 92.12 (2008): 1636-1641.

Wong, Tien, et al. "The natural history and prognosis of neovascular age-related macular degeneration: a systematic review of the literature and meta-analysis." *Ophthalmology* 115.1 (2008): 116-126.

Group, Collaborative Normal-Tension Glaucoma Study. "Comparison of glaucomatous progression between untreated patients with normal-tension glaucoma and patients with therapeutically reduced intraocular pressures."*American Journal of Ophthalmology* 126.4 (1998): 487-497.

Leibowitz, Howard M., et al. "The Framingham Eye Study monograph: an ophthalmological and epidemiological study of cataract, glaucoma, diabetic retinopathy, macular degeneration, and visual acuity in a general population of 2631 adults, 1973-1975." *Survey of Ophthalmology* 24.Suppl (1979): 335-610.

Kass, Michael A., et al. "The Ocular Hypertension Treatment Study: a randomized trial determines that topical ocular hypotensive medication delays or prevents the onset of primary open-angle glaucoma." *Archives of Ophthalmology* 120.6 (2002): 701-713.

Quigley, Harry A., Gregory R. Dunkelberger, and W. Richard Green. "Chronic human glaucoma causing selectively greater loss of large optic nerve fibers." *Ophthalmology* 95.3 (1988): 357-363.

Leske, M. Cristina. "The epidemiology of open-angle glaucoma: a review." *American Journal of Epidemiology* 118.2 (1983): 166-191.

Hodapp, Elizabeth, Richard K. Parrish, and Douglas R. Anderson. *Clinical Decisions in Glaucoma.* Mosby Inc, 1993.

Grant, W. Morton, and Joseph F. Burke. "Why do some people go blind from glaucoma?" *Ophthalmology* 89.9 (1982): 991-998.

Foster, Paul J., et al. "The definition and classification of glaucoma in prevalence surveys." *British journal of ophthalmology* 86.2 (2002): 238-242.

Leske, M. Cristina, et al. "Factors for glaucoma progression and the effect of treatment: the early manifest glaucoma trial." *Archives of ophthalmology* 121.1 (2003): 48-56.

Alvarado, Jorge, Collin Murphy, and Richard Juster. "Trabecular meshwork cellularity in primary open-angle glaucoma and nonglaucomatous normals." *Ophthalmology* 91.6 (1984): 564-579.

Flammer, Josef. "The vascular concept of glaucoma." *Survey of ophthalmology* 38 (1994): S3-S6.

Weinreb, Robert N., and Peng Tee Khaw. "Primary open-angle glaucoma." *The Lancet* 363.9422 (2004): 1711-1720.

Leske, M. Cristina, et al. "Predictors of long-term progression in the early manifest glaucoma trial." *Ophthalmology* 114.11 (2007): 1965-1972.

Wandel, Thaddeus. "Treatment of glaucoma." U.S. Patent No. 5,807,302. 15 Sep. 1998.

Migdal, Clive, Walter Gregory, and Roger Hitchings. "Long-term functional outcome after early surgery compared with laser and medicine in open-angle glaucoma." *Ophthalmology* 101.10 (1994): 1651-1657.

Watson, Peter G., and Ian Grierson. "The place of trabeculectomy in the treatment of glaucoma." *Ophthalmology* 88.3 (1981): 175-196.

Beebe, Walter E., et al. "The use of Molteno implant and anterior chamber tube shunt to encircling band for the treatment of glaucoma in keratoplasty patients." *Ophthalmology* 97.11 (1990): 1414-1422.

Sherwood, M. B., et al. "Drainage tube implants in the treatment of glaucoma following penetrating keratoplasty." *Ophthalmic surgery* 24.3 (1993): 185-189.

Cozean, Colette, et al. "Laser surgical procedures for treatment of glaucoma." U.S. Patent No. 5,865,831. 2 Feb. 1999.

Jampel, Henry D., et al. "Perioperative complications of trabeculectomy in the collaborative initial glaucoma treatment study (CIGTS)." *American Journal of Ophthalmology* 140.1 (2005): 16-22.

Watson, P. G., et al. "The complications of trabeculectomy (a 20-year follow-up)." *Eye* 4.3 (1990): 425-438.

Adamis, Anthony P., et al. "Increased vascular endothelial growth factor levels in the vitreous of eyes with proliferative diabetic retinopathy."*American Journal of Ophthalmology* 118.4 (1994): 445-450.

Joussen, Antonia M., et al. "A central role for inflammation in the pathogenesis of diabetic retinopathy." *The FASEB Journal* 18.12 (2004): 1450-1452.

Danis, Ronald P., and Matthew D. Davis. "Proliferative Diabetic Retinopathy." *Diabetic Retinopathy*. Humana Press, 2008. 29-65.

Avery, Robert L., et al. "Intravitreal bevacizumab (Avastin) in the treatment of proliferative diabetic retinopathy." *Ophthalmology* 113.10 (2006): 1695-1705.

Klein, Barbara EK, et al. "Diabetic retinopathy: assessment of severity and progression." *Ophthalmology* 91.1 (1984): 10-17.

López, Fernando, et al. "Diabetic retinopathy treatment." *European Ophthalmic Review* (2007): 68-70.

Ferris, Frederick L. "How effective are treatments for diabetic retinopathy?." *Jama* 269.10 (1993): 1290-1291.

Spaide, Richard F., and Yale L. Fisher. "Intravitreal bevacizumab (Avastin) treatment of proliferative diabetic retinopathy complicated by vitreous hemorrhage." *Retina* 26.3 (2006): 275-278

Mason, John O., Peter A. Nixon, and Milton F. White. "Intravitreal injection of bevacizumab (Avastin) as adjunctive treatment of proliferative diabetic retinopathy." *American Journal of Ophthalmology* 142.4 (2006): 685-688.

Elman, Michael J., et al. "Intravitreal ranibizumab for diabetic macular edema with prompt versus deferred laser treatment: three-year randomized trial results." *Ophthalmology* 119.11 (2012): 2312-2318.

Crawford, Talia N., et al. "Diabetic retinopathy and angiogenesis." *Current Diabetes Reviews* 5.1 (2009): 8-13..

Yam, Jason CS, and Alvin KH Kwok. "Update on the treatment of diabetic retinopathy." *Hong Kong Medical Journal* 13.1 (2007): 46.

CHAPTER 4:

Kern, David E. *Curriculum Development for Medical Education: A Six-Step Approach*. JHU Press, 1998.

Lempp, Heidi, and Clive Seale. "The hidden curriculum in undergraduate medical education: qualitative study of medical students' perceptions of teaching." *BMJ* 329.7469 (2004): 770-773.

Nandi, P. L., et al. "Undergraduate medical education: comparison of problem-based learning and conventional teaching." *Hong Kong Medical Journal* 6.3 (2000): 301-306.

Moffat, Katrina J., et al. "First year medical student stress and coping in a problem-based learning medical curriculum." *Medical Education* 38.5 (2004): 482-491.

Bannerman, Robert H., John Burton, and Wen-Chieh Ch'en. "Traditional medicine and health care coverage: a reader for health administrators and practitioners." *Traditional Medicine and Health Care Coverage: A Reader for Health Administrators and Practitioners.* (1983).

Nicholls, Phillip A. *Homoeopathy and the Medical Profession.* Croom Helm Ltd, 1988.

Tovey, Philip, et al. "Patient assessment of effectiveness and satisfaction with traditional medicine, globalized complementary and alternative medicines, and allopathic medicines for cancer in Pakistan." *Integrative Cancer Therapies* 4.3 (2005): 242-248.

Semmes, Clovis E. "Nonmedical illness behavior: a model of patients who seek alternatives to allopathic medicine." *Journal of Manipulative and Physiological Therapeutics* 13.8 (1990): 427-436.

Johnson, Shirley M., and Margot E. Kurtz. "Perceptions of philosophic and practice differences between US osteopathic physicians and their allopathic counterparts." *Social Science & Medicine* 55.12 (2002): 2141-2148.

Sackett, David L. "Evidence-based medicine." *Seminars in Perinatology.* Vol. 21. No. 1. WB Saunders, 1997.

Evidence-Based Medicine Working Group. "Evidence-based medicine. A new approach to teaching the practice of medicine." *Jama* 268.17 (1992): 2420.

Haynes, R. Brian. "What kind of evidence is it that Evidence-Based Medicine advocates want health care providers and consumers to pay attention to?." *BMC Health Services Research* 2.1 (2002): 1.

Bates, David W., et al. "Ten commandments for effective clinical decision support: making the practice of evidence-based medicine a reality." *Journal of the American Medical Informatics Association* 10.6 (2003): 523-530.

Coomarasamy, Arri, and Khalid S. Khan. "What is the evidence that postgraduate teaching in evidence based medicine changes anything? A systematic review." *BMJ* 329.7473 (2004): 1017.

Feinstein, Alvan R., and Ralph I. Horwitz. "Problems in the 'evidence' of 'evidence-based medicine'." *The American Journal of Medicine* 103.6 (1997): 529-535.

Isaacs, David, and Dominic Fitzgerald. "Seven alternatives to evidence based medicine." *BMJ* 319.7225 (1999): 1618.

Maynard, Alan. "Evidence-based medicine: an incomplete method for informing treatment choices." *The Lancet* 349.9045 (1997): 126-128.

Straus, Sharon E., and Finlay A. McAlister. "Evidence-based medicine: a commentary on common criticisms." *Canadian Medical Association Journal* 163.7 (2000): 837-841.

Timmermans, Stefan, and Aaron Mauck. "The promises and pitfalls of evidence-based medicine." *Health Affairs* 24.1 (2005): 18-28.

Grahame-Smith, David. "Evidence based medicine: Socratic dissent." *BMJ* 310.6987 (1995): 1126.

Lipsky, Martin S., and Lisa K. Sharp. "From idea to market: the drug approval process." *The Journal of the American Board of Family Practice* 14.5 (2001): 362-367.

Wood, Alastair JJ. "A proposal for radical changes in the drug-approval process." *New England Journal of Medicine* 355.6 (2006): 618-623.

Rutherford, Elizabeth M. "FDA and Privatization-The Drug Approval Process, The." *Food & Drug LJ* 50 (1995): 203.

Zuckerman, Diana M., Paul Brown, and Steven E. Nissen. "Medical device recalls and the FDA approval process." *Archives of Internal Medicine* 171.11 (2011): 1006-1011.

Friedman, Michael A., et al. "The safety of newly approved medicines: do recent market removals mean there is a problem?." *Jama* 281.18 (1999): 1728-1734.

Dohrman, Amanda J. "Rethinking and Restructuring the FDA Drug Approval Process in Light of the Vioxx Recall." *J. Corp. L.* 31 (2005): 203.

Avorn, Jerry. "Paying for drug approvals—who's using whom?." *New England Journal of Medicine* 356.17 (2007): 1697-1700.

DiMasi, Joseph A., Ronald W. Hansen, and Henry G. Grabowski. "The price of innovation: new estimates of drug development costs." *Journal of Health Economics* 22.2 (2003): 151-185.

Adams, Christopher P., and Van V. Brantner. "Estimating the cost of new drug development: is it really $802 million?." *Health Affairs* 25.2 (2006): 420-428.

Dickson, Michael, and Jean Paul Gagnon. "Key factors in the rising cost of new drug discovery and development." *Nature Reviews Drug Discovery* 3.5 (2004): 417-429.

Gieringer, Dale H. "Safety and Efficacy of New Drug Approval, The." *Cato J.* 5 (1985): 177.

Dickson, Michael, and Jean Paul Gagnon. "The cost of new drug discovery and development." *Discovery Medicine* 4.22 (2009): 172-179.

Klein, Donald F. "The flawed basis for FDA post-marketing safety decisions: the example of anti-depressants and children." *Neuropsychopharmacology* 31.4 (2006): 689-699.

Kulynych, Jennifer. "Will FDA Relinquish the Gold Standard for New Drug Approval-Redefining Substantial Evidence in the FDA Modernization Act of 1997." *Food & Drug LJ* 54 (1999): 127.

Bean, Melissa Marie. "Fatal Flaws in the Food and Drug Administration's Drug-Approval Formula." *Utah L. Rev.* (2003): 881.

Proudfoot, John R. "The evolution of synthetic oral drug properties." *Bioorganic & Medicinal Chemistry Letters* 15.4 (2005): 1087-1090.

Patridge, Eric, et al. "An analysis of FDA-approved drugs: natural products and their derivatives." *Drug Discovery Today* (2015).

Ganesan, A. "The impact of natural products upon modern drug discovery." *Current opinion in chemical biology* 12.3 (2008): 306-317.

Newman, David J., and Gordon M. Cragg. "Natural Products as Sources of New Drugs over the Last 25 Years." *Journal of Natural Products* 70.3 (2007): 461-477.

Siahpush, Mohammad. "Postmodern values, dissatisfaction with conventional medicine and popularity of alternative therapies." *Journal of Sociology* 34.1 (1998): 58-70.

Siahpush, Mohammad. "Why do people favour alternative medicine?." *Australian and New Zealand Journal of Public Health* 23.3 (1999): 266-271.

White, Philip. "What can general practice learn from complementary medicine?" *BJGP* 50.459 (2000): 821-823.

Meeker, William C. "Public demand and the integration of complementary and alternative medicine in the US health care system." *Journal of Manipulative and Physiological Therapeutics* 23.2 (2000): 123-126.

Robinson, Anske, and M. R. McGrail. "Disclosure of CAM use to medical practitioners: a review of qualitative and quantitative studies." *Complementary Therapies in Medicine* 12.2 (2004): 90-98.

Wetzel, Miriam S., David M. Eisenberg, and Ted J. Kaptchuk. "Courses involving complementary and alternative medicine at US medical schools." *Jama* 280.9 (1998): 784-787.

CHAPTER 5:

Prensky, Marc. "How to teach with technology: Keeping both teachers and students comfortable in an era of exponential change." *Emerging Technologies for Learning* 2.4 (2007): 40-46.

Ashley, Steven. "Cutting costs and time with DFMA." *Mechanical Engineering* 117.3 (1995): 74.

Collins, Jannette. "Education Techniques for Lifelong Learning: Giving a PowerPoint Presentation: The Art of Communicating Effectively 1." *Radiographics* 24.4 (2004): 1185-1192.

Chandra, Ranjit Kumar. "Nutrition and the immune system: an introduction." *The American journal of clinical nutrition* 66.2 (1997): 460S-463S.

Wilkens, Lynne R., and James Lee. *Nutritional Epidemiology*. John Wiley & Sons, Ltd, 1998.

Who, Joint, and FAO Expert Consultation. "Diet, nutrition and the prevention of chronic diseases." *World Health Organ Tech Rep Ser* 916.i-viii (2003).

Ames, Bruce N. "Low micronutrient intake may accelerate the degenerative diseases of aging through allocation of scarce micronutrients by triage." *Proceedings of the National Academy of Sciences* 103.47 (2006): 17589-17594.

Stratton, Rebecca J., Ceri J. Green, and Marinos Elia. *Disease-Related Malnutrition: An Evidence-Based Approach to Treatment*. Cabi, 2003.

Strong, Kathleen, et al. "Preventing chronic diseases: how many lives can we save?." *The Lancet* 366.9496 (2005): 1578-1582.

Kumar, Neeraj. "Neurologic presentations of nutritional deficiencies." *Neurologic Clinics* 28.1 (2010): 107-170.

Goodwin, James S. "Social, psychological and physical factors affecting the nutritional status of elderly subjects: separating cause and effect." *The American Journal of Clinical Nutrition* 50.5 (1989): 1201-1209.

Prasad, Ananda S. "Zinc deficiency." *BMJ* 326.7386 (2003): 409-410.

Butterworth, Roger F. "Metal toxicity, liver disease and neurodegeneration." *Neurotoxicity Research* 18.1 (2010): 100-105.

Doudoroff, Peter, et al. "Bio-assay methods for the evaluation of acute toxicity of industrial wastes to fish." *Sewage and Industrial Wastes* (1951): 1380-1397.

Liao, Chung-Min, et al. "Acute toxicity and bioaccumulation of arsenic in tilapia (Oreochromis mossambicus) from a blackfoot disease area in Taiwan." *Environmental Toxicology and Chemistry* 18.4 (2003): 252-259.

Fu, Li-Jie, Robert E. Staples, and Ralph G. Stahl. "Assessing acute toxicities of pre- and post-treatment industrial wastewaters with Hydra attenuata: A comparative study of acute toxicity with the fathead minnow, Pimephales promelas." *Environmental Toxicology and Chemistry* 13.4 (1994): 563-569.

Botham, P. A. "Acute systemic toxicity—prospects for tiered testing strategies." *Toxicology in Vitro* 18.2 (2004): 227-230.

Mayer, Foster Lee, and Mark R. Ellersieck. *Manual of Acute Toxicity: Interpretation and Data Base for 410 Chemicals and 66 Species of Freshwater Animals.* Washington, DC: US Department of the Interior, Fish and Wildlife Service, 1986.

Todd, Andrew C., et al. "Unraveling the chronic toxicity of lead: an essential priority for environmental health." *Environmental Health Perspectives* 104. Suppl 1 (1996): 141.

Ajani, Jaffer A., et al. "Comprehensive criteria for assessing therapy-induced toxicity." *Cancer Investigation* 8.2 (1990): 147-159.

Barnes, J. M., and F. A. Denz. "Experimental Methods Used in Determining Chronic Toxicity A Critical Review." *Pharmacological Reviews* 6.2 (1954): 191-242.

Ospina-Tascon, Gustavo, et al. "Effects of fluids on microvascular perfusion in patients with severe sepsis." *Intensive Care Medicine* 36.6 (2010): 949-955.

Sakr, Yasser, et al. "Persistent microcirculatory alterations are associated with organ failure and death in patients with septic shock." *Critical Care Medicine-Baltimore* 32.9 (2004): 1825-1831.

McDonagh, Paul, and Jason Y. Hokama. "Microvascular perfusion and transport in the diabetic heart." *Microcirculation* 7.3 (2000): 163-181.

Bodí, Vicente, et al. "Microvascular perfusion 1 week and 6 months after myocardial infarction by first-pass perfusion cardiovascular magnetic resonance imaging." *Heart* 92.12 (2006): 1801-1807.

Levy, Bernard I., et al. "Impaired tissue perfusion a pathology common to hypertension, obesity, and diabetes mellitus." *Circulation* 118.9 (2008): 968-976.

Bateman, Ryon M., and Keith R. Walley. "Microvascular resuscitation as a therapeutic goal in severe sepsis." *Critical Care* 9.Suppl 4 (2005): S27.

De Backer, Daniel, et al. "Microcirculatory alterations: potential mechanisms and implications for therapy." *Ann Intensive Care* 1.1 (2011): 27.

CHAPTER 6:

Thompson, Gary D. "Consumer demand for organic foods: what we know and what we need to know." *American Journal of Agricultural Economics* 80.5 (1998): 1113-1118.

Dimitri, Carolyn, and Catherine Greene. "Recent growth patterns in the US organic foods market." *Agriculture Information Bulletin* 777 (2000).

Winter, Carl K., and Sarah F. Davis. "Organic foods." *Journal of Food Science* 71.9 (2006): R117-R124.

Larue, Bruno, et al. "Consumer response to functional foods produced by conventional, organic, or genetic manipulation." *Agribusiness* 20.2 (2004): 155-166.

Crinnion, Walter J. "Organic foods contain higher levels of certain nutrients, lower levels of pesticides, and may provide health benefits for the consumer." *Alternative Medicine Review* 15.1 (2010): 4-13.

Jones, Peter, et al. "Retailing organic foods." *British Food Journal* 103.5 (2001): 358-365.

Magnusson, Maria K., et al. "Choice of organic foods is related to perceived consequences for human health and to environmentally friendly behaviour." *Appetite* 40.2 (2003): 109-117.

Saba, Anna, and Federico Messina. "Attitudes towards organic foods and risk/benefit perception associated with pesticides." *Food Quality and Preference* 14.8 (2003): 637-645.

Hino, Akihiro. "Safety assessment and public concerns for genetically modified food products: the Japanese experience." *Toxicologic Pathology* 30.1 (2002): 126-128.

Liu, Chenglin. "Is USDA Organic a Seal of Deceit: The Pitfalls of USDA Certified Organics Produced in the United States, China and Beyond." Stan. J. Int'l L. 47 (2011): 333.

Winter, Carl K., and Sarah F. Davis. "Organic foods." *Journal of Food Science* 71.9 (2006): R117-R124.

Thompson, P., et al. "Livestock welfare product claims: The emerging social context." *Journal of Animal Science* 85.9 (2007): 2354-2360.

Boland, Michael, and Ted Schroeder. "Marginal value of quality attributes for natural and organic beef." *Journal of Agricultural and Applied Economics* 34.01 (2002): 39-49.

Joint, F. A. O., *WHO Expert Committee on Food Additives, and World Health Organization*. "Evaluation of certain food additives and contaminants: thirtieth report of the Joint FA." (1987).

Concon, Jose M. *Food Toxicology. Part A: Principles and concepts; Part B: Contaminants and additives*. Marcel Dekker Inc., 1988.

Furia, Thomas E. *CRC Handbook of Food Additives*. Vol. 1. CRC press, 1973.

Joint, F. A. O. "Evaluation of certain food additives." *24th Report of the Joint FAO/WHO Expert Committee on Food Additives*. 1980.

Ashley, David VM. "Factors affecting the selection of protein and carbohydrate from a dietary choice." *Nutrition Research* 5.5 (1985): 555-571.

Steffen, Lyn M., et al. "Associations of whole-grain, refined-grain, and fruit and vegetable consumption with risks of all-cause mortality and incident coronary artery disease and ischemic stroke: the Atherosclerosis Risk in Communities (ARIC) Study." *The American Journal of Clinical Nutrition* 78.3 (2003): 383-390.

Dicke, W. K., H. A. Weijers, and J. H. Kamer. "Coeliac Disease The Presence in Wheat of a Factor Having a Deleterious Effect in Cases of Coeliac Disease." *Acta Paediatrica* 42.1 (1953): 34-42.

Pereira, Mark A., et al. "Effect of whole grains on insulin sensitivity in overweight hyperinsulinemic adults." *The American Journal of Clinical Nutrition* 75.5 (2002): 848-855.

Liu, Simin, et al. "A prospective study of dietary glycemic load, carbohydrate intake, and risk of coronary heart disease in US women." *The American Journal of Clinical Nutrition* 71.6 (2000): 1455-1461.

Jenkins, D. J., et al. "Glycemic index of foods: a physiological basis for carbohydrate exchange." *The American Journal of Clinical Nutrition* 34.3 (1981): 362-366.

Oh, Kyungwon, et al. "Carbohydrate intake, glycemic index, glycemic load, and dietary fiber in relation to risk of stroke in women." *American Journal of Epidemiology* 161.2 (2005): 161-169.

Gaby, Alan R. "Adverse effects of dietary fructose." *Alternative Medicine Review* 10.4 (2005): 294.

Biesalski, H-K. "Meat as a component of a healthy diet—are there any risks or benefits if meat is avoided in the diet?." *Meat Science* 70.3 (2005): 509-524.

Salmeron, Jorge, et al. "Dietary fat intake and risk of type 2 diabetes in women." *The American Journal of Clinical Nutrition* 73.6 (2001): 1019-1026.

Sacks, Frank M., and Martijn Katan. "Randomized clinical trials on the effects of dietary fat and carbohydrate on plasma lipoproteins and cardiovascular disease." *The American Journal of Medicine* 113.9 (2002): 13-24.

McGuire, M. A., and M. K. McGuire. "Conjugated linoleic acid (CLA): A ruminant fatty acid with beneficial effects on human health." *Journal of Animal Science* 77.E-Suppl (2000): 1-8.

Wood, J. D., et al. "Effects of fatty acids on meat quality: a review." *Meat Science* 66.1 (2004): 21-32.

Risérus, Ulf, Walter C. Willett, and Frank B. Hu. "Dietary fats and prevention of type 2 diabetes." *Progress in Lipid Research* 48.1 (2009): 44-51.

Bonanome, A., et al. "virgin olive oil." *European Journal of Clinical Investigation* 35.7 (2005): 421-424.

Dansinger, Michael L., et al. "Comparison of the Atkins, Ornish, Weight Watchers, and Zone diets for weight loss and heart disease risk reduction: a randomized trial." *Jama* 293.1 (2005): 43-53.

Enos, William F., Robert H. Holmes, James Beyer. "Coronary Disease Among United States Soldiers Killed in Action in Korea." *Jama.* 1953; 152(12):1090-1093.

McNamara, J. Judson, Mark A. Molot, John F. Stremple, Robert T. Cutting. "Coronary Artery Disease in Combat Casualties in Vietnam." *Jama.* 1971; 216(7):1185-1187.

Goldberg, P., M. C. Fleming, and E. H. Picard. "Multiple sclerosis: decreased relapse rate through dietary supplementation with calcium, magnesium and vitamin D." *Medical Hypotheses* 21.2 (1986): 193-200.

Rath, Matthias, and Aleksandra Niedzweicki. "Nutritional Supplement Program Halts Progression of Early Coronary Atherosclerosis Documented by Ultrafast Computerized Tomography." *Journal of Applied Nutrition* 48.3 (1996): 67-78.

Lieberman, Shari, Nancy Pauling Bruning, and Nancy Bruning. *The Real Vitamin and Mineral Book: A Definitive Guide to Designing Your Personal Supplement Program.* Penguin, 2007.

Greenwald, Peter, et al. "Clinical trials of vitamin and mineral supplements for cancer prevention." *The American Journal of Clinical Nutrition* 85.1 (2007): 314S-317S.

Willett, Walter C., and Meir J. Stampfer. "What vitamins should I be taking, doctor?." *New England Journal of Medicine* 345.25 (2001): 1819-1824.

Fortmann, Stephen P., et al. "Vitamin and mineral supplements in the primary prevention of cardiovascular disease and cancer: an updated systematic evidence review for the US Preventive Services Task Force." *Annals of Internal Medicine* 159.12 (2013): 824-834.

Ley, Sylvia H., et al. "Prevention and management of type 2 diabetes: dietary components and nutritional strategies." *The Lancet* 383.9933 (2014): 1999-2007.

Yehuda, Shlomo, Sharon Rabinovitz, and David I. Mostofsky. "Essential fatty acids are mediators of brain biochemistry and cognitive functions." *Journal of Neuroscience Research* 56.6 (1999): 565-570.

Yehuda, Shlomo. "Omega-6/omega-3 ratio and brain-related functions." (2003): 37-56.

Yehuda, Shlomo, et al. "Fatty acids and brain peptides." *Peptides* 19.2 (1998): 407-419.

Yehuda, Shlomo, Sharon Rabinovitz, and David I. Mostofsky. "Mixture of essential fatty acids lowers test anxiety." *Nutritional Neuroscience* 8.4 (2005): 265-267.

CHAPTER 7:

Ayres, Robert U. "Toxic heavy metals: materials cycle optimization." *Proceedings of the National Academy of Sciences* 89.3 (1992): 815-820.

BJ Alloway. Heavy metals in soils. *Springer Science & Business Media*, 1995.

Chowdhury, Badrul Alam, and Ranjit Kumar Chandra. "Biological and health implications of toxic heavy metal and essential trace element interactions." *Progress in Food & Nutrition Science* 11, no. 1 (1986): 55-113.

Inoue, K. I. "Heavy Metal Toxicity." *J Clinic Toxicol* S 3 (2013): 2161-0495.

Graeme, Kimberlie A., and Charles V. Pollack. "Heavy metal toxicity, part I: arsenic and mercury." *The Journal of Emergency Medicine* 16.1 (1998): 45-56.

Depledge, M. H., J. M. Weeks, and P. Bjerregaard. "Heavy metals." *Handbook of Ecotoxicology* (1994): 543-569.

Lorscheider, Fritz L., Murray J. Vimy, and Anne O. Summers. "Mercury exposure from" silver" tooth fillings: emerging evidence questions a traditional dental paradigm." *The FASEB Journal* 9.7 (1995): 504-508.

Björkman, L., G. Sandborgh-Englund, and J. Ekstrand. "Mercury in saliva and feces after removal of amalgam fillings." *Toxicology and Applied Pharmacology* 144.1 (1997): 156-162.

Stenman, Svante, and Leif Grans. "Symptoms and differential diagnosis of patients fearing mercury toxicity from amalgam fillings." *Scandinavian Journal of Work, Environment & Health* (1997): 59-63.

Fung, Yiu K., and Michael P. Molvar. "Toxicity of mercury from dental environment and from amalgam restorations." *Journal of Toxicology: Clinical Toxicology* 30.1 (1992): 49-61.

Aposhian, H. V., et al. "Urinary mercury after administration of 2, 3-dimercaptopropane-1-sulfonic acid: correlation with dental amalgam score." *The FASEB Journal* 6.7 (1992): 2472-2476.

Berglund, A. "Estimation by a 24-hour study of the daily dose of intra-oral mercury vapor inhaled after release from dental amalgam." *Journal of Dental Research* 69.10 (1990): 1646-1651.

Mutter, Joachim, et al. "Mercury and autism: accelerating evidence." *Neuroendocrinol Lett* 26.5 (2005): 439-446.

Soden, Sarah E., et al. "24-hour provoked urine excretion test for heavy metals in children with autism and typically developing controls, a pilot study." *Clinical Toxicology* 45.5 (2007): 476-481.

Aposhian, H. Vasken, et al. "Mobilization of heavy metals by newer, therapeutically useful chelating agents." *Toxicology* 97.1 (1995): 23-38.

Blaurock-Busch, Eleonor, Omnia R. Amin, and Thanaa Rabah. "Heavy metals and trace elements in hair and urine of a sample of arab children with autistic spectrum disorder." *Maedica* (Buchar) 6 (2011).

Crinnion, Walter J. "The benefits of pre-and post-challenge urine heavy metal testing: Part 1." *Alternative Medicine Review* 14.1 (2009): 3-9.

Brodkin, Elizabeth, et al. "Lead and mercury exposures: interpretation and action." *Canadian Medical Association Journal* 176.1 (2007): 59-63.

Chernecky, Cynthia C., and Barbara J. Berger. Laboratory tests and diagnostic procedures. *Elsevier Health Sciences*, 2007.

Graeme, Kimberlie A., and Charles V. Pollack. "Heavy metal toxicity, part I: arsenic and mercury." *The Journal of Emergency Medicine* 16.1 (1998): 45-56.

Aposhian, H. Vasken, et al. "Mobilization of heavy metals by newer, therapeutically useful chelating agents." *Toxicology* 97.1 (1995): 23-38.

Catsch, Alexander, A-E. Harmuth-Hoene, and David P. Mellor. The chelation of heavy metals. Vol. 70. *Pergamon*, 1979.

Lamas, Gervasio A., et al. "Effect of disodium EDTA chelation regimen on cardiovascular events in patients with previous myocardial infarction: the TACT randomized trial." *Jama* 309.12 (2013): 1241-1250.

Casdorph, H. Richard. "EDTA chelation therapy, efficacy in arteriosclerotic heart disease." *J Holistic Med* 3.1 (1981): 53-59.

Chisolm, J. Julian. "The use of chelating agents in the treatment of acute and chronic lead intoxication in childhood." *The Journal of Pediatrics* 73.1 (1968): 1-38.

Patrick, Lyn. "Lead toxicity, a review of the literature. Part I: exposure, evaluation, and treatment." *Alternative Medicine Review* 11.1 (2006): 2-23.

George, Graham N., et al. "Mercury binding to the chelation therapy agents DMSA and DMPS and the rational design of custom chelators for mercury." *Chemical Research in Toxicology* 17.8 (2004): 999-1006.

Vasken Aposhian, H., et al. "Human studies with the chelating agents, DMPS and DMSA." *Journal of Toxicology: Clinical Toxicology* 30.4 (1992): 505-528.

Aaseth, Jan, et al. "Treatment of mercury and lead poisonings with dimercaptosuccinic acid and sodium dimercaptopropanesulfonate. A review." *Analyst* 120.3 (1995): 853-854.

CHAPTER 8

Rajaram, Sri-Sujanthy, et al. "Enhanced external counter pulsation (EECP) as a novel treatment for restless legs syndrome (RLS): a preliminary test of the vascular neurologic hypothesis for RLS." *Sleep Medicine* 6.2 (2005): 101-106.

Barsheshet, Alon, et al. "The effects of external counter pulsation therapy on circulating endothelial progenitor cells in patients with angina pectoris." *Cardiology* 110.3 (2007): 160-166.

Erdling, André, et al. "Enhanced external counter pulsation in treatment of refractory angina pectoris: two year outcome and baseline factors associated with treatment failure." *BMC Cardiovascular Disorders* 8.1 (2008): 1.

Manchanda, Aarush, and Ozlem Soran. "Enhanced external counterpulsation and future directions: step beyond medical management for patients with angina and heart failure." *Journal of the American College of Cardiology* 50.16 (2007): 1523-1531.

Werner, Dierk, et al. "Pneumatic external counterpulsation: a new noninvasive method to improve organ perfusion." *The American Journal of Cardiology* 84.8 (1999): 950-952.

Rajaram, Sri-Sujanthy, Peter Rudzinskiy, and Arthur S. Walters. "Enhanced external counter pulsation (EECP) for restless legs syndrome (RLS): preliminary negative results in a parallel double-blind study." *Sleep Medicine* 7.4 (2006): 390-391.

Taguchi, Isao, et al. "Effects of Enhanced External Counterpulsation on Hemodynamics and Its Mechanism-Relation to Neurohumoral Factors." *Circulation Journal* 68.11 (2004): 1030-1034.

Urano, Hisashi, et al. "Enhanced external counterpulsation improves exercise tolerance, reduces exercise-induced myocardial ischemia and improves left ventricular diastolic filling in patients with coronary artery disease." *Journal of the American College of Cardiology* 37.1 (2001): 93-99.

Lawson, William E., et al. "Three-year sustained benefit from enhanced external counterpulsation in chronic angina pectoris." *The American Journal of Cardiology* 75.12 (1995): 840-841.

Arora, Rohit R., et al. "Effects of enhanced external counterpulsation on Health-Related Quality of Life continue 12 months after treatment: a substudy of the Multicenter Study of Enhanced External Counterpulsation." *Journal of Investigative Medicine* 50.1 (2002): 25-32.

Akhtar, Mateen, et al. "Effect of external counterpulsation on plasma nitric oxide and endothelin-1 levels." *The American Journal of Cardiology* 98.1 (2006): 28-30.

Cai, Dawei, Ruiliang Wu, and Ying Shao. "Experimental study of the effect of external counterpulsation on blood circulation in the lower extremities." *Clinical and Investigative Medicine* 23.4 (2000): 239.

Werner, Dierk, et al. "Accelerated reperfusion of poorly perfused retinal areas in central retinal artery occlusion and branch retinal artery occlusion after a short treatment with enhanced external counterpulsation." *Retina* 24.4 (2004): 541-547.

Han, Jing Hao, et al. "Preliminary findings of external counterpulsation for ischemic stroke patient with large artery occlusive disease." *Stroke* 39.4 (2008): 1340-1343.

Feldman, Arthur M. "Enhanced external counterpulsation: mechanism of action." *Clinical Cardiology* 25.S2 (2002): 11-15.

Zhen-sheng, Z. H. E. N. G. "The past, present and future of external counterpulsation." *Journal of Sun Yat-Sen University (Medical Sciences)* 6 (2006): 003.

Bregman, David, Bruce L. Hanson, and Sidney Wolvek. "Apparatus for aiding and improving the blood flow in patients." U.S. Patent No. 4,080,958. 28 Mar. 1978.

Coletti, R. H., et al. "Abdominal Counterpulsation (AC)-A New Concept in Circulatory Assistance." *ASAIO Journal* 28.1 (1982): 563-566.

Werner, Dierk, et al. "Changes in ocular blood flow velocities during external counterpulsation in healthy volunteers and patients with atherosclerosis." *Graefe's Archive for Clinical and Experimental Ophthalmology* 239.8 (2001): 599-602.

Lin, Wenhua, et al. "External counterpulsation augments blood pressure and cerebral flow velocities in ischemic stroke patients with cerebral intracranial large artery occlusive disease." *Stroke* 43.11 (2012): 3007-3011.

Froschermaier, Stefan E., et al. "Enhanced external counterpulsation as a new treatment modality for patients with erectile dysfunction." *Urologia Internationalis* 61.3 (1999): 168-171.

Hilz, M. J., et al. "Enhanced external counterpulsation improves skin oxygenation and perfusion." *European Journal of Clinical Investigation* 34.6 (2004): 385-391.

Werner, Dierk, et al. "Enhanced external counterpulsation: a new technique to augment renal function in liver cirrhosis." *Nephrology Dialysis Transplantation* 20.5 (2005): 920-926.

Jungehuelsing, G. J., et al. "Does external counterpulsation augment mean cerebral blood flow in the healthy brain? Effects of external counterpulsation on middle cerebral artery flow velocity and cerebrovascular regulatory response in healthy subjects." *Cerebrovascular Diseases* 30.6 (2010): 612-617.

Levenson, Jaime, et al. "Effects of enhanced external counterpulsation on carotid circulation in patients with coronary artery disease." *Cardiology* 108.2 (2007): 104-110.

Jewell, C. W., et al. "Enhanced external counterpulsation is a regenerative therapy." *Frontiers in Bioscience* (Elite edition) 2 (2009): 111-121.

Lipson, Charles S., and James E. Nicholson. "Pressure cycle for stimulating blood circulation in the limbs." U.S. Patent No. 3,901,221. 26 Aug. 1975.

Stiller, M. J., et al. "A portable pulsed electromagnetic field (PEMF) device to enhance healing of recalcitrant venous ulcers: a double-blind, placebo-controlled clinical trial." *British Journal of Dermatology* 127.2 (1992): 147-154.

Assiotis, Aggelos, Nick P. Sachinis, and Byron E. Chalidis. "Pulsed electromagnetic fields for the treatment of tibial delayed unions and nonunions. A prospective clinical study and review of the literature." *Journal of Orthopaedic Surgery and Research* 7.1 (2012): 1.

Glazer, Paul Andrew, and Lian Clamen Glazer. "Electricity: the history and science of bone growth stimulation for spinal fusion." *Orthop J Harvard Med School Online* 4 (2002): 63-67.

Saltzman, Charles, Andrew Lightfoot, and Annunziato Amendola. "PEMF as treatment for delayed healing of foot and ankle arthrodesis." *Foot & Ankle International* 25.11 (2004): 771-773.

Piatkowski, Joachim, Simone Kern, and Tjalf Ziemssen. "Effect of BEMER magnetic field therapy on the level of fatigue in patients with multiple sclerosis: a randomized, double-blind controlled trial." *The Journal of Alternative and Complementary Medicine* 15.5 (2009): 507-511.

Hug, Kerstin, and Martin Röösli. "Therapeutic effects of whole-body devices applying pulsed electromagnetic fields (PEMF): A systematic literature review." *Bioelectromagnetics* 33.2 (2012): 95-105.

Pretorius, Leon, and Dietmar H. Winzker. "Biomedical technology: a case study of forecasting in pulsed electro magnetic field therapy." Technology Management for Global Economic Growth (PICMET), *2010 Proceedings of PICMET'10:*. IEEE, 2010.

Beamer, Sharon L., Ken W. Grant, and Brian E. Walden. "Hearing aid benefit in patients with high-frequency hearing loss." *Journal-American Academy of Audiology* 11.8 (2000): 429-437.

Tysarczyk-Niemeyer, Georg. "New noninvasive pQCT devices to determine bone structure." *J Jpn Soc Bone Morphom* 7 (1997): 97-105.

Milewski, Stanisław, et al. "Effect of pulsed electromagnetic fields on hematological and biochemical blood indices and milk production in sheep."Electr. J. Polish Agric. Univ., Vet. *Med* 4.2 (2001).

Bohn, Wolfgang, Lorenzo Hess, and Ralph Burger. "The effects of the 'physical BEMER® vascular therapy', a method for the physical stimulation of the vasomotion of precapillary microvessels in case of impaired microcirculation, on sleep, pain and quality of life of patients with different clinical pictures on the basis of three scientifically validated scales." *Journal of Complementary and Integrative Medicine* 10.Suppl (2013): S5-S12.

Gazurek, D., and K. Spodaryk. "BEMER 3000 on Ratings of Perceived Exertion." *Biol. Sport* 25.2 (2008): 147-165.

Gleim, Peter. "Apparatus for modulating perfusion in the microcirculation of the blood." U.S. Patent Application No. 13/145,963.

Říhová, Blanka, et al. "Synergistic effect of EMF–BEMER-type pulsed weak electromagnetic field and HPMA-bound doxorubicin on mouse EL4 T-cell lymphoma." *Journal of Drug Targeting* 19.10 (2011): 890-899.

Walther, Markus, et al. "Effects of weak, low-frequency pulsed electromagnetic fields (BEMER type) on gene expression of human mesenchymal stem cells and chondrocytes: an in vitro study." *Electromagnetic Biology and Medicine* 26.3 (2007): 179-190.

Gleim, Peter, and Rainer Klopp. "Device for generating a pulsed electromagnetic field with pulse control." U.S. Patent No. 8,216,121. 10 Jul. 2012.

Tennant, Jerry. *Healing is Voltage: The Handbook*. publisher not identified, 2010.

McMakin, Carolyn R., and James L. Oschman. "Visceral and somatic disorders: Tissue softening with frequency-specific microcurrent." *The Journal of Alternative and Complementary Medicine* 19.2 (2013): 170-177.

Oschman, James L. *Energy Medicine in Therapeutics and Human performance*. Edinburgh, Scotland: Butterworth Heinemann, 2003.

McMakin, C. "Non-pharmacologic treatment of neuropathic pain using frequency specific microcurrent." *Pain Practitioner* 20.3 (2010): 68-73.

McMakin, Carolyn R., and James L. Oschman, "Visceral and Somatic Disorders: Tissue Softening with Frequency-Specific Microcurrent." *JACM*, 19: 2, 2013. *Yoga Sudha* 20: 170-177.

McMakin, C. *Frequency Specific Microcurrent in Pain Management*. Edinburgh: Churchill Livingstone. (2011).

Feig, Stephen A., et al. "Summary of the American college for advancement in medicine November 2004 conference on emerging concepts in immunology." *Evidence-Based Complementary and Alternative Medicine* 2.1 (2005): 121.

Chen, George, and Kuo Chiang. "Method and apparatus for applying microcurrent to eyes." U.S. Patent Application No. 10/853,242.

Baxter, Chad, et al. "1506 Choice and outcomes of alternative therapies in patients with interstitial cystitis (IC) and chronic pelvic pain (CPP)." *The Journal of Urology* 183.4 (2010): e580.

McMakin, Carolyn. "Microcurrent therapy in the treatment of fibromyalgia." *Fibromyalgia Syndrome: A Practitioner's Guide to Treatment*. Edinburgh: Churchill Livingstone (2003): 179-206.

Rossen, Joel. *Introduction to Microcurrent and Guide to Its Greatest Effectiveness*. Pengrove, Carliff (1989).

McMakin, Carolyn R., Walter M. Gregory, and Terry M. Phillips. "Cytokine changes with microcurrent treatment of fibromyalgia associated with cervical spine trauma." *Journal of Bodywork and Movement Therapies* 9.3 (2005): 169-176.

Chaikin, Laurie, et al. "Microcurrent stimulation in the treatment of dry and wet macular degeneration." *Clinical ophthalmology* (Auckland, NZ) 9 (2015): 2345.

Sw, Mean Ear, and Side Eff. "Detailed summary about FSM."

Liu, Haitao, et al. "Metanx and Early Stages of Diabetic RetinopathyMetanx and Early Diabetic Retinopathy." *Investigative Ophthalmology & Visual Science* 56.1 (2015): 647-653.

Shevalye, Hanna, et al. "Metanx alleviates multiple manifestations of peripheral neuropathy and increases intraepidermal nerve fiber density in Zucker diabetic fatty rats." *Diabetes* 61.8 (2012): 2126-2133.

CHAPTER 10:

Lindvall, Olle, Zaal Kokaia, and Alberto Martinez-Serrano. *Stem Cell Therapy for Human Neurodegenerative Disorders–How to Make it Work*. (2004): S42-S50.

Segers, Vincent FM, and Richard T. Lee. "Stem-cell therapy for cardiac disease." *Nature* 451.7181 (2008): 937-942.

Murphy, J. Mary, et al. "Stem cell therapy in a caprine model of osteoarthritis." *Arthritis & Rheumatism* 48.12 (2003): 3464-3474.

Strauer, Bodo E., and Ran Kornowski. "Stem cell therapy in perspective." *Circulation* 107.7 (2003): 929-934.

Marx, Robert E. "Platelet-rich plasma (PRP): what is PRP and what is not PRP?." *Implant Dentistry* 10.4 (2001): 225-228.

Weibrich, Gernot, et al. "Growth factor levels in platelet-rich plasma and correlations with donor age, sex, and platelet count." *Journal of Cranio-Maxillofacial Surgery* 30.2 (2002): 97-102.

Dugrillon, A., et al. "Autologous concentrated platelet-rich plasma (cPRP) for local application in bone regeneration." *International Journal of Oral and Maxillofacial Surgery* 31.6 (2002): 615-619.

Sampson, Steven, Michael Gerhardt, and Bert Mandelbaum. "Platelet rich plasma injection grafts for musculoskeletal injuries: a review." *Current Reviews in Musculoskeletal Medicine* 1.3-4 (2008): 165-174.

Alsousou, J., et al. "The biology of platelet-rich plasma and its application in trauma and orthopaedic surgery A REVIEW OF THE LITERATURE." *Journal of Bone & Joint Surgery, British Volume* 91.8 (2009): 987-996.

Hall, Michael P., et al. "Platelet-rich Plasma: Current Concepts and Application in Sports Medicine." *Journal of the American Academy of Orthopaedic Surgeons* 17.10 (2009): 602-608.

Bianco, Paolo, and Pamela Gehron Robey. "Stem cells in tissue engineering." *Nature* 414.6859 (2001): 118-121.

Kern, Susanne, et al. "Comparative analysis of mesenchymal stem cells from bone marrow, umbilical cord blood, or adipose tissue." *Stem cells* 24.5 (2006): 1294-1301.

Lee, Oscar K., et al. "Isolation of multipotent mesenchymal stem cells from umbilical cord blood." *Blood* 103.5 (2004): 1669-1675.

Wagner, Wolfgang, et al. "Comparative characteristics of mesenchymal stem cells from human bone marrow, adipose tissue, and umbilical cord blood." *Experimental Hematology* 33.11 (2005): 1402-1416.

Sample, CD45. "Isolation of human mesenchymal stem cells: bone marrow versus umbilical cord blood." *Haematologica* 86 (2001): 10.

Secco, Mariane, et al. "Multipotent stem cells from umbilical cord: cord is richer than blood!." *Stem Cells* 26.1 (2008): 146-150.

Baker, Paul S., and Gary C. Brown. "Stem-Cell Therapy in Retinal Disease." *Current Opinion in Ophthalmology* 20.3 (2009): 175-181.

Tibbetts, Michael D., et al. "Stem cell therapy for retinal disease." *Current Opinion in Ophthalmology* 23.3 (2012): 226-234.

Ahmad, Iqbal. "Stem cells: new opportunities to treat eye diseases." *Investigative Ophthalmology & Visual Science* 42.12 (2001): 2743-2748.

Levin, Leonard A., et al. "Stem cell therapy for ocular disorders." *Archives of Ophthalmology* 122.4 (2004): 621-627.

Meyer, Jason S., et al. "Optic vesicle-like structures derived from human pluripotent stem cells facilitate a customized approach to retinal disease treatment." *Stem Cells* 29.8 (2011): 1206-1218.

Johnson, Thomas V., et al. "Neuroprotective effects of intravitreal mesenchymal stem cell transplantation in experimental glaucoma." *Investigative Ophthalmology & Visual Science* 51.4 (2010): 2051-2059.

Rowland, Teisha J., David E. Buchholz, and Dennis O. Clegg. "Pluripotent human stem cells for the treatment of retinal disease." *Journal of Cellular Physiology* 227.2 (2012): 457-466.